THE CAUSE OF

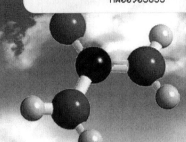

BREAST CANCER REVEALED

And Science-Based Method to Keep it a...S.L.E.E.P.

JACQUIE HART

The information contained in this book is the result of experience and research of the author or other sources referenced in this book. The nutritional, therapeutic and hormonal advice is in no way intended as medical advice or as a substitute for medical counseling. Not all the information, statements, advice, opinions, or material referenced have been evaluated by the FDA and should not be relied upon to diagnose, treat, cure or prevent any condition or disease. Before beginning any therapeutic regimen, including diet, exercise and supplementation, it is advisable to seek the advice of a physician. Your physician should be aware of all medical conditions that you may have, as well as the medications and supplements you are taking. The author accepts no responsibility or liability for the use of any information or material contained in this book.

TABLE OF CONTENTS

INTRODUCTION

PART I
WAKING UP

PART II
HORMONE TESTING AND PLANNING

PART III
TAKING ACTION

INTRODUCTION

Wouldn't it be great if you knew what causes breast cancer? Perhaps, if you did, you could significantly decrease your chance of getting it. Hi, I am Jacquie Hart. I wrote this testimony as proof that breast cancer can be prevented. I didn't realize it before, but I found out that scientists already know what causes 75% of breast cancer. They *do* know the reason why breast cancer cells grow and surprisingly, there *is* a way to prevent this growth. I was so amazed when I was able to get rid of my own breast lumps, I did a lot of research to uncover the facts behind why I was able to shrink them, so I could help other women do the same.

With the help of my doctor, I have proved that being proactive works. By finding out the main cause of breast cancer, I was able to intercept it and so can you. I used my doctor's protocol, which I termed the S.L.E.E.P. Method, to eliminate the cause. You will get to see my pictures that prove it!

If you work the S.L.E.E.P. Method into your life as well as share it with others, you will not only decrease your risk, but you will be decreasing the risk for our society as a whole and future generations. By spreading the word to other women, together we can make a difference.

Maybe you have struggled with breast cancer already. Maybe you are afraid it could happen to you and want to do everything to prevent it. Either way, through perseverance, you have the ability to do this method. We can only put this terminal enemy to sleep if we wake up to its cause. Unfortunately, the enemy is not something we can see with our own eyes, yet we are exposed to it daily.

After we learn what the cause is, complacency gets put aside and it becomes a simple choice to make a plan of action. Knowledge, planning and action- that is all it takes and that is how I've divided up this book.

I have put together for you the most recent breast cancer research, along with my personal healing experience in one easy to understand, action-oriented how-to book. I've included the latest information from medical books, doctors, scientific research, articles, and testimonies into three parts to help fill the knowledge gap around this deadly disease.

In today's society, we find that the medical community and natural community are at odds over cures and techniques. In this book, I bridge the gap between technical knowledge of the medical world with science-backed natural alternative solutions. These two worlds no longer have to fight. In fact, you may be surprised how much the medical world is actually utilizing natural solutions and supplements. The medical and natural communities can work together to stop this unrelenting disease!

Part I will bring you the science and knowledge behind breast cancer's main cause and from where it's coming.

In Part II, you will find the best tools to use in finding your personal health status. This is where you will discover if you are one of many people at risk for this type of breast cancer as well as where your risks lie. I also bring you tips on finding the best doctor for your situation. In this chapter, you get everything ready to take action.

Part III is the action phase. This is the best part, which I am really excited about. I've coined an easy to remember name that women can use to help keep them on track and to spread the word. My hope is that your determination will be contagious. You can help put a majority of breast cancer to rest through this awareness and my **S.L.E.E.P. Method**.

Each letter in the S.L.E.E.P. Method stands for one step to keep breast cancer asleep. Each step includes methods that are backed by scientific evidence and follow only one premise - to remove from your body the one thing that causes 75% or more of breast cancer. This is the only text where you can find one complete compilation of scientifically backed removal strategies for preventing breast cancer. The S.L.E.E.P. Method incorporates diet, lifestyle, household, personal care, and birth control choices along with scientifically proven supplements. Medical research that supports steps in this method is crucial, so I have included footnotes and references.

If we can stop putting this one thing into our body in the first place and then get it out of our body, we can win. This is where you will gear up to battle against this one thing, which you will find out about very soon.

The S.L.E.E.P. Method can be tailored to your own individual situation. I've put these removal strategies in clear and simple terms so you can choose what is best for you. I'll give you the "perfect" scenario with these five steps. You can do some, or all of it as you desire, however, your chances of prevention or recovery are higher and quicker if you attempt to do them all. Even if you decide only to do parts of the S.L.E.E.P. Method, well, it's better to do a little bit o' something than a whole lot of nothin'! If this one thing is not an issue for you, these steps include scientifically-backed recommendations for other causes too, so read on!

Besides my own testimony, you will get to hear about some successful, invigorating, real-life testimonies of women, who follow this protocol or parts thereof. Perhaps these stories will be the flame to light your fire or to support your journey toward prevention or healing. There is even an easy to follow, realistic action guide that will help you get started. When you're finished with this method, you will have an opportunity to discuss your journey with other women, share ideas, and find products that work with it.

Several doctors' books were referenced in writing this book. Together, these doctors' facts and risk reduction strategies are the tools I used for healing and are the foundations of the S.L.E.E.P. methodology. The five steps in the S.L.E.E.P. Method incorporate proven scientific methods recommended from Bruce Rind, M.D.; Susan Love, M.D.; John R. Lee, M.D.; Jonathan V. Wright, M.D.; Lane Lenard, Ph.D.; David Brownstein, M.D.; and Joseph Mercola, D.O. These doctors are leaders in the health industry, both mainstream and integrative. Along with proven research and clinical success through their own practices, these five methods used alone and together have been proven to be effective against breast cancer.

Susan Love, M.D., MBA is a retired breast cancer surgeon who has devoted her professional life to being an activist in the eradication of breast cancer. She is a trusted source to women worldwide through her books and Foundation website (Dr. Susan Love Research Foundation). She authored *Dr. Susan Love's Breast Book*, which was termed "the bible for women with breast cancer" by The New York Times. In her book, she explains in an understandable way, the science behind and options for breast cancer treatment. She has also pioneered the way for breast cancer research by launching an internet solution that partners women to scientists.

Jonathan V. Wright, M.D. is a medical doctor who expanded knowledge of the natural human hormonal system by copying nature. In 1982, he was the first physician in North America to prescribe bio-identical hormone replacement and was also the first to publish a book on hormone replacement in 1997. He has been practicing since 1970, founded Tahoma Clinic near Seattle, Washington in 1973 (www.TahomaClinic.com) and has authored or co-authored fourteen books on natural therapies, including three about bio-identical hormones. Together with Lane Lenard, Ph.D., he wrote the book *Stay Young & Sexy With Bio-identical Hormones: The Science Explained*, the most comprehensive book available to date on this topic.

John R. Lee, M.D. started publishing books on conventional hormone replacement therapy (HRT) in the 1990s. Although Dr. Lee died in October 2003, his work lives on in his best-selling books, tapes, and the Official Website of John R. Lee, M.D. (www.JohnLeeMD.com). He was an international authority and pioneer in the use of natural progesterone cream and hormone balance. His book, *What Your Doctor May Not Tell You About Breast Cancer*, became the cornerstone and inspiration of my book.

Joseph Mercola, D.O. has been an osteopathic doctor since 1982 and currently practices alternative medicine. He has become popular over the internet with his website and newsletter, where he offers information and supplements for natural healing. His website is touted as the most popular natural healing website. He has written two books that made *The New York Times* best sellers' list.

Bruce Rind, M.D. is one of the leading integrative medical doctors in the Washington metropolitan area and my personal doctor. He has been practicing integrative medicine since 1985. He is an expert in women's health and has developed a few of his own supplements to help women's issues. His office utilizes thermography detection as an additional tool for identifying problem areas in the breast. He utilizes both natural and medical knowledge to best suit the patient's needs.

I would like to recognize several people for being a personal inspiration for completing this book: Craig Ballantyne and Michael Masterson (Mark Ford) for being my virtual mentors through their online newsletter *Early To Rise*; my pastor, Barry White, for strengthening my faith and providing clarity; Dr. Rind and his team for showing me first-hand how breast cancer can be prevented; Lee and Sally Kroon for spending time reading and providing feedback to ensure accuracy in parts of this book. Emily Wright for editing word after word. Lastly, my mom and husband for years of editing assistance, encouragement and listening to my revelations.

PART I

WAKING UP

Chapter 1

CAUSE OF BREAST CANCER

An Obscure Reality

The reality of breast cancer is difficult to face when it touches our lives personally. We do our routine examine every year. We check ourselves to make sure there are no new lumps. Then one day it happens. We find an unusual lump. That's when we start to get scared. That's when we might start to do research.

At least that's what happened to me. The only reason I even started to care about breast cancer is because I found lumps in my breasts. Oh, and my younger brother found breast lumps too. I didn't ever think it could happen to me, much less my brother.

As an indoor environmental consultant, I investigate causes of health issues in people's homes. I see first-hand how disturbed people become when they have an illness, and are not able to figure out how or why it started. They will pay any amount of money and do everything in their power to find out the cause.

It happened to me the first time I was told there was an unusual, extra lump in my body and told there was nothing I could do. That was when I found a cyst in my breast that was confirmed through ultrasound. At least with home investigations, I am able to help people narrow down what the cause of their allergies or illness might be. It is a shame that it is hasn't been quite so simple with breast cancer.

Years after the cyst, I got that same devastating feeling when I found out I had a dominant lump in my left breast. Luckily, the lump didn't turn out to be cancer, or at least not detectable by the mammogram. That lump could have turned into breast cancer if I hadn't gotten rid of it. I wouldn't have known I had the lump, much less that I could do something about it, if it weren't for the methods recommended by my proactive doctor.

After using his science-backed alternative methods, I was able to heal my own body. I was so amazed at the results that I decided to find out what was going on and perhaps reveal this protocol to others. Just maybe, I could help others do the same thing. Well, I didn't need to be a scientist to do some research, analyze details, and assemble it all together.

You see, the main reason why the cause of breast cancer remains elusive is because there are many parts contributing to it and these parts together as a whole haven't been given a title or a name. The science is available and there are doctors who understand why it is caused. It can even be found in a handful of books, but it is hidden in them as if it is a big secret. What is the reason? The answer is three-fold. First, it takes analyzing the little details in breast cancer science to arrive at the big picture. Second, making a big conclusion about all the details also encompasses liability for anyone who does it. Third, there is no money to be made, at least at this time, behind its cause.

So I'm writing this book to give breast cancer's cause a name, draw the appropriate conclusion and explain the details. Someone ought to do it and the time is now! I was astonished that in this day and age, there has been no big announcement of breast cancer's cause, with the number of women being diagnosed (232,340 US women in 2013). Taking into consideration the population increase, breast cancer incidence has increased four-fold since 1970[1]. The rising trend keeps rising. If it gets higher every year, as it has, we may be heading for a pandemic.

Breast cancer has become the second most common cause of death for middle-aged women, but most of us don't think that we will ever get it.

---

[1] Siegel, Zou, Jemal, 2014 *The Linacre Quarterly* 81 (3).

Unfortunately, this belief, combined with obscure information, causes us to do very little to prevent it until we are affected by it.

Many times when we find out we have breast cancer or a lump, we are told there is not much we can do to make it go away and are only given a few methods we can use to prevent it. However, as I found out, there is a way to prevent it in the first place, to shrink cancer tumors![2]

If you think about it, modern medicine utilizes radiation and drugs such as chemotherapy and tamoxifen to shrink cancer. A study by the National Surgical Adjuvant Breast and Bowel Project found an 80% reduction in tumor size and that 36% of the tumors disappeared completely using chemotherapy.[3] This is without surgery! Are radiation and drugs the only methods able to shrink cancer? Actually, there are many safe methodologies that are being utilized to shrink tumors and benign lumps. These methods are just not publicized. Scientists have discovered breast cancer's main cause and it can be prevented and even stopped!

The Cause Revealed

Scientists have known the leading reason for breast cancer since it was proven in studies dating back to the 1960s. Professor Henry Lemon discovered that women were more likely to survive long-term after breast cancer tumor removal if they had more estriol in their urine specimens, rather than estrone and estradiol.[4] This signified that one of the estrogens, estriol, was protective and the other two estrogens were growth promoters. These two estrogens, estrone and estradiol, are the root cause of breast cancer tumor growth.

------

[2] Baker, Sherry Jan 2013 *Health Sciences* "Proof: Breast cancer cells can revert to normal without drugs".

[3] Fisher B et al. 1998 *Journal of the National Cancer Institute* "Tamoxifen for prevention of breast cancer: Report of The National Surgical Adjuvant Breast and Bowel Project P-1 study".

[4] Lemon, HM Apr. 1969 Cancer "Endocrine influences on human mammary cancer formation. A critique".

Researchers at pharmaceutical companies utilize this knowledge of estrogens and have been trying to find breast cancer cures they can patent. Some drugs have been developed and patented, but unfortunately, they may not always be effective or they may include bad side effects. Once you get breast cancer, if you are put on these drugs, that's when you find out what the drugs are doing. They are opposing estrogen in the breast! These drugs themselves are one of five ways that plainly displays breast cancer's cause.

I couldn't believe it, but the answer also lies right there in breast cancer and hormone books and websites ... 75% of breast cancer is caused by ... excess ESTROGENS. In many breast cancer books, one section will say scientists and doctors don't know the original cause of breast tumors, but right there in the next section they are talking about breast cancer **estrogen receptors** being found on a large majority of tumors and drugs that treat them. This is crazy! They do know that 75% of tumors grow due to these estrogen receptors within the tumor, combined with an estrogenic environment. This is a second example that demonstrates estrogen is at the heart of breast cancer.

Then there are even quotes from real medical doctors. Here is what Dr. Susan Love, a well-known retired breast cancer surgeon, has to say about hormones and breast cancer in her book *Dr. Susan Love's Breast Book*:

"They (hormones) *most definitely are a major influence on, if not a cause of breast cancer."*[5]

If we look, it's right there in front of us. I found five areas where we can see the clear truth. If we can understand that breast cancer's cause is just this one thing ...estrogenic factors ... then maybe, we get ahead of the breast cancer nightmare and keep it asleep before it grows!

---

[5] Susan M Love, MD *Dr. Susan Love's Breast Book* 2010 p.150

Estrogen Receptor-Positive Tumors as Proof

Acquiring an understanding of how estrogen receptors work reveals that estrogen is indeed involved in breast cancer. 75% of breast cancer cells grow due to excess estrogens, which has been proven by tumor biopsies taken from patients. Scientists found out that tumors had hormone receptors on them. Ever since the mid-1980s, doctors have been performing biopsies when a patient is diagnosed with breast cancer, to determine if the tumor is estrogen/progesterone receptor-positive. They use a core needle to remove tumor tissue and then they test that piece of tumor for multiple characteristics to determine what kind of cancer the patient has. Scientists and doctors have found that 75% of breast cancer tumors test positive for extra estrogen/progesterone receptors.[6]

In order to understand how estrogen and progesterone receptors affect breast cancer, we need to understand how hormones and receptors work together. Hormones move around the body by traveling in the blood stream. A hormone receptor is a cell protein that binds to hormones as they pass by in the blood. Normal breast cells have hormone receptors.

Estrogen receptors help to promote breast development in cells during teenage years and pregnancy. When there is excessive estrogen and insufficient progesterone, a decrease in receptor sensitivity occurs. It is well known that women with low progesterone have trouble conceiving and have a much higher risk of getting breast cancer. [7]

For some breast cancer patients, both estrogen and progesterone receptors increase, yet the reasons are not yet clear why *progesterone* receptors increase. One hypothesis could be that the cell responds to decreased estrogen receptor sensitivity by making more estrogen receptors. Since one of progesterone's functions is to restore normal

---

[6] ww5.komen.org, and www.webmd.com
[7] Cowan LD et al. Aug 1981 *Am J Epidemiol* "Breast cancer incidence in women with a history of progesterone deficiency".

sensitivity of estrogen receptors, the cell then proceeds to make more progesterone receptors in order to attempt to increase progesterone.

Just this year, it was proven that when progesterone is restored, estrogen receptor sensitivity is also restored and the number of receptors normalize.[8] This detailed study was just what was needed to prove one of progesterone's roles in controlling actions of estrogen and its role in breast cancer!

When estrogens bind to estrogen receptors in a cancer cell, the estrogens interact with genes of tumor cells and cause the cells to grow. For this reason, scientists know if a tumor tests estrogen/progesterone receptor-positive, the tumor has grown due to excess estrogen.

There is no intention on my part to paint a bad picture of estrogen here. Estrogens exist for a reason. They are not really *bad* unless you have too much. Estrogens exist to promote cell growth for the breast during puberty and pregnancy and in the uterus to carry a baby. Too much estrogen causes the regular system of cell development and growth to be disrupted, causing an overproduction of normal-appearing cells. Basically, estrogen in excess causes cells to replicate. So there you have it!

Drugs as Proof

Not only do tumor biopsies demonstrate that estrogen grows breast cancer tumors, but the drugs given to estrogen receptor-positive women, reveal it. In fact, the very drugs that were developed to prevent breast cancer are antagonists to estrogens. Drugs like *tamoxifen, raloxifene, fulvestrant*, and *goserelin* are the most commonly prescribed drugs for breast cancer patients with estrogen or progesterone receptor-positive tumors. Guess what these drugs do?

---

[8] Mohammed, Hisham, et al. 2015 *Nature* "Progesterone receptor modulates ER-α action in breast cancer".

They interrupt the estrogen receptor and inevitably stop estrogen from its normal process of cell replication. With the use of the drug *goserelin,* production of estrogen in the ovaries is stopped altogether.

Tamoxifen has been shown to reduce the risk of breast cancer recurrence by 29 to 38%.[9] Women who test positive for atypical cells (not yet cancerous) in their milk duct cells are known to have a 200% relative risk for breast cancer.[10] For prevention, women who had biopsies showing atypical cells were treated with *tamoxifen* for five years by Dr. David Page. There were 86% fewer subsequent breast cancers over the period of the study than those who had no treatment.[11] Other randomized studies have shown this effect.

These estrogen interrupting drugs such as tamoxifen are called *anti-estrogens.* Take note that these do not block progesterone. Progesterone is not what causes cell division.[12] Progesterone in normal amounts opposes estrogen and acts as an antagonist to it. If progesterone is low and estrogen is high, cell replication will occur. Anti-estrogen drugs attempt to block estrogen receptors, which paralyze the receptor and prevent it from triggering events that result in cell division. Hence, the second way that demonstrates 75% of breast cancer is caused by estrogen. The first is patient tumor biopsies. The second is the very drugs prescribed to prevent breast cancer.

[9] Allred DC et al. Apr 2012 *J Clin Oncol* "Adjuvant tamoxifen reduces subsequent breast cancer in women with estrogen receptor-positive ductal carcinoma in situ: a study based on NSABP protocol B-24".

[10] Page DL, et al. Jan 2003 *Lancet* "Atypical lobular hyperplasia as a unilateral predictor of breast cancer risk: a retrospective cohort study".

[11] 1988 *New England Journal of Medicine* "Early Breast Cancer Collaborative Trialists' Group, Effects of adjuvant tamoxifen and of cytotoxic therapy on mortality in early breast cancer: An overview of 61 randomized trials among 28,896 women".

[12] B. Formby and T.S. Wiley 1998, The Sansum Medical Research Foundation in Santa Barbara, CA, *Annals of Clinical and Laboratory Science* Estrogen added to breast cancer cell cultures activated the oncogene (cancer-causing gene) *bcl-2*, whereas progesterone activated the cancer-protective gene called *p53*.

With these anti-estrogen drugs, the medical industry is what is driving the cure for breast cancer. Sadly, all of these drugs come with major side effects such as blood clotting problems, strokes and uterine cancer. Tamoxifen actually stimulates the ovaries to make more estrogen while blocking estrogen receptors in the breast. It is in fact, acting like an estrogen in other organs such as the uterus and bone. Also, these drugs do not have a high levels of effectiveness, so scientists are trying to improve them. Scientists are working on killing cancer directly, too (there's more information on this later in Part I).

Human Study as Proof

Not only do tumor biopsies and breast cancer drugs prove that breast cancer is caused by estrogen, there are even human drug trials verifying it. A very significant study event happened in mid-2002. A large, double-blind placebo-controlled clinical trial of 161,000 women in the US by NIH, intended to last nine years, was cut short. The trial was for women aged 50 to 79 years of age who were being treated for postmenopausal symptoms and uterine removal. The Women's Health Initiative (WHI) study had two components. The main portion that was being treated for postmenopausal symptoms was halted after 5.2 years. Why did scientists stop this portion of the study early? To everyone's surprise, it was because 26% of women had an increase in breast cancer and increase of cardiovascular events from the drug that was being tested.[13]

This drug combined horse estrogen (Premarin) and a synthetic progesterone-like synthetic drug (medroxyprogesterone or MPA). *Prempro* was the resulting combined drug. Horse estrogen has many differences from human estrogen, and the synthetic progesterone may act to oppose horse estrogen to prevent endometrial cancer (hence the reason why pharmaceutical companies added it), but it acts like estrogen in other aspects such as cell replication.

---

[13]Anderson GL et al 2003 *J Amer Med Assoc* "Effects of estrogen plus progestin on gynecologic cancers and associated diagnostic procedures: The Women's Health Initiative randomized trial".

Incidentally, the second arm of the study which was on women who no longer had uteruses and were given horse urine estrogen pills (*Premarin*), was also terminated early after seven years due to the significant increased risk of stroke. This medication also had a previous history of causing endometrial cancer, but that risk would obviously be gone simply by the fact that these women had no uterus. It is interesting to note that breast cancer did not increase with *Premarin* medication, but slightly declined. This could be partially due to fact that these women did not have ovaries to produce estrogen themselves but it also goes to show that not all hormones affect the human body in the same way. Some hormones may have an affinity to the uterus, cervix, or thyroid. The synthetic version of progesterone (medroxyprogesterone or MPA) was a trigger toward breast cancer. The natural horse estrogen was not a trigger for breast cancer.

After the first portion of the study was stopped and the news had gotten out about the increase in breast cancer, people stopped taking *Prempro*. Subsequently, there was a significant decrease in breast cancer across our population. There are conflicting reports on the actual decrease percentage in breast cancer rate. According to www.breastcancer.org, breast cancer decreased by 2% per year from 1999 to 2005. Dr. Joseph Mercola's website reports as much as 36% decline in total deaths of women in the US from 1990 to 2005. Other books cite an 18% decrease in year one after the study in 2003. Whatever the number, there was enough of an *increase* in incidence during the study and *decrease* in incidence and deaths afterwards to prove that synthetic hormone was indeed causing breast cancer in hundreds of thousands of women. In 2013, The National Cancer Institute made a statement that the combined estrogen/progestin HRT is associated with "approximately a 26% increase in incidence of invasive breast cancer".[14]

---

[14] www.cancer.gov/types/breast/hp/breast-prevention-pdq

22

After this one significant study event, Dr. Jonathan Wright assembled a graph based on reviews published in 2007.[15] These reviews documented breast cancer incidence, estrogen receptor-positive tumors and HRT prescriptions. Utilizing the data from these reviews, Dr. Wright's chart illustrates a direct linear correlation between estrogen receptor-positive (ER+) tumors and HRT prescriptions use.

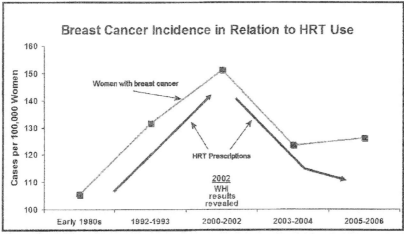

Figure 1-1. The incidence of breast cancer among women aged 45 and older has risen and fallen over the last 3 decades in direct correlation with the number of prescriptions of conventional "hormone" replacement (HRT) therapy (Premarin® + Provera®). Looking at these data, scientists have declared it "the smoking gun" that proves that HRT causes breast cancer.

Adapted from Ravdin PM, et al. *N Engl J Med.* 2007;356:1670-1674 and Glass AG, et al. *J. Natl. Cancer Inst.* 2007;99:1152-1161.

Stay Young & Sexy with Bio-Identical Hormone Replacement by Jonathan V. Wright, MD and Lane Lenard, PhD 2010 p.2. Reprinted with permission from www.smart-publications.com

This trial is just one of many previous and ongoing human studies demonstrating that estrogenic factors are what cause breast cancer.

---

[15] Ravdin, PM et al. 2007 N Engl J Med "The decrease in breast-cancer incidence in 2003 in the United States", and Glass AG et al. 2007 J Natl Cancer Inst "Breast Cancer incidence, 1980-2006: Combined roles of menopausal therapy, screening mammography and estrogen receptor status".

Cancer Cell Origin and Growth as Proof

On a molecular level, scientists have been able to find explanations as to why an original cell mutates, or changes. These theories on how they form in the first place are also related to estrogen!

There are two critical elements needed for cancer to start in the first place and then grow. First, the original cell must undergo a mutation in its DNA. This DNA mutation modifies how the cell behaves in its environment, but this mutation alone may not be enough to cause tumor growth.

The second element involves the environment the cell is in. In a breast cancer scenario, the fat cells, immune cells, blood cells and lymph all surround the breast cancer cell. If this environment (also called the stroma) is all well behaved, the cancer will not grow. But if the surrounding cells stimulate or even tolerate the tumor cell, they can help create mutated cells and growth. The question is, what makes DNA mutate and what makes an environment not well behaved?

A majority of researchers support one of two of the following theories that answer the question of DNA mutation, both of which relate to estrogen. In a scientific statement in 2009, The Endocrine Society speaks of the "somatic mutation theory".[16] This is when a cell undergoes growth, month after consistent month of exposure to estrogenic activity, during times when there is meant to be low amounts. This estrogenic activity happens with frequency over the course of a person's lifetime due to exposure to carcinogens such as radiation, chemicals in foods or environmental pollutants. Eventually the cell changes its DNA code, which is referred to as a mutation. The mutation is an altered set of instructions that is different from our

---

[16] Diamanti-Kandarakis, Evanthia et al. Jun 2009 *Endocr* "Endocrine-Disrupting Chemicals: An Endocrine Society Scientific Statement".

original program, so to speak. This mutation is what can make a cancer cell.

However, it takes repeated exposures to carcinogens and many cell alterations in genes to get cancer. It is not typically due to just one cell or a one-time exposure. For example, we know cigarette smoking causes lung cancer. It is not caused by smoking just one or two cigarettes. In fact, our body has repair mechanisms to correct abnormal DNA changes but sometimes the repair mechanisms fail themselves.

A second explanation of cancer cell origin is the "tissue organization field theory".[6] This is where the surrounding tissue of cells is architecturally changed by estrogens, which eventually changes or causes the cells to mutate.

There is a third theory discussed by Dr. Michael Galiltzer in Suzanne Somers *Knockout* called the "low oxygen theory".[5] In this theory, toxicity accumulates in the body over time, which may be caused by internal or external factors. Regular cells use oxygen to create energy. The toxic factors deplete respiratory enzymes, so the cells can no longer use oxygen. Since these cells can no longer use oxygen, they mutate to accommodate their situation and start utilizing sugar to create energy. Cancer cells are those very cells. They do not use oxygen; they use sugar for their energy to grow. Sugar is known to be estrogenic![17]

Wherever and however these mutated cells start, our mutated cells make copies of themselves as we age. This would explain why they accumulate over time. Eventually we end up as a bunch of photo copies of errors, which explains why cancer risk increases with age.

You can see there are many possible reasons why cancer cells originate and replicate. It seems reasonable that all of these theories are correct.

---

[17] Wairagu, PM et al 2015 *Cancer Biol Ther* "Insulin priming effect on estradiol-induced breast cancer metabolism and growth".

When I investigate mold in peoples' homes, many times, the mold growth is happening due to several reasons and moisture sources. There is not always just one source. If we understand that cancer cells exist in our bodies, then we can plainly see that the most important question is *not* how they form, but what sources cause them to grow. Science has unequivocally answered that most important question: excess estrogen or estrogenic factors!

Quotes as Proof

Not only do cancer cell growth theories, studies, current drug treatment and tumor biopsies prove that excess estrogens are the main cause of breast cancer, but organizations believe it too. Here is what they have to say:

The Breast Cancer Institute says this in their 2007 edition of the *Breast Cancer Prevention Institute Online Booklet*:

"In general, most breast cancer risk factors, other than inherited genes and chemical or radiation injury to cells, are related to how much estrogen a woman is exposed to in her lifetime and how early she matures her breast lobules to Type 3".[18]

The National Cancer Institute reports that 75% of breast tumors test positive for estrogen/progesterone receptors. Sometimes breast cancers that are estrogen positive can test negative for progesterone.[19]

The Endocrine Society in their 2009 Scientific Statement states this:

"In summary, exposure to estrogen throughout a woman's life, including the period of intrauterine development, is a risk factor for the development of breast cancer. The increased incidence of breast cancer noted during the last 50 years may have been caused, in part, by

---

[18] www.bcpinstitute.org/booklet4.htm *Breast Cancer Prevention Institute Online Booklet* Dr. Angela Lanfranchi and Dr. Joel Brind 2005 Chapter 2
[19] www.cancer.gov

exposure of women to estrogen-mimicking chemicals that have been released into the environment from industrial and commercial sources." [20]

WebMD also states "about 75% of breast cancers are ER positive. They grow in response to the hormone estrogen." [21]

Susan G. Komen states on their website, "Most (about two out of three) breast cancers are hormone receptor-positive."[22]

Conclusion

As you can see with these five facts, there is too much history and evidence that proves excess estrogen or excess stimulation of estrogen and the lack of estrogen-opposing hormones is the cause of growth of most breast cancers. So why hasn't anyone made this announcement? There are a few reasons why as I mentioned before. The most relevant is that there is a cumulative effect of estrogen sources that build-up in our body. Many studies only study one aspect such as one chemical or one birth control pill or they test blood serum, which is not where chemical-like estrogens are stored. Also, some doctors may not be aware of the studies behind this truth or may be afraid to make a statement due to liability and fear of losing their credentials. In effect, there is liability associated with it.

If you look carefully, however, which we will do in the next chapter and Part III, you will see that each individual source is linked to breast cancer. The accumulation of estrogen-stimulating sources, most significantly of chemicals, metals, pesticides, sugar intake and patentable hormones in our bodies, are together what causes breast cancer.

---

[20] www.endocrine.org Diamanti-Kandarakis, Evanthia et al. *Endocrine Disrupting Chemicals: An Endocrine Society Scientific Statement* p. 17

[21] www.webmd.com/breast -ccancerbreast-cancer-types-er-positive-her2-positive

[22] ww5.komen.org/BreastCancer/TumorCharacteristics.html

Lucky or unlucky for me, I don't have any medical licenses, so I can lay it all on the line. It was convincing enough for me when I saw first-hand my personal case study as well as others'. I was amazed at what can happen when excess estrogens are removed from the body and the impact on the body from patentable hormones. I have thermography photographs to demonstrate my case and you will get to see those in Part II. It is due time to wake everybody up to the cause!

Eventually, pharmaceutical companies may come up with a pill or patch that works to block estrogens without side effects. In the meantime, we can stop the onslaught of estrogens we are putting into our bodies! With this guide in your hands, you can choose to control tumor cell growth by taking control of these sources.

Chapter 2

CAUSE OF ESTROGEN INCREASE

Rising Estrogen

Our bodies are in an invisible war against hormones...and we don't even realize it! I didn't know it either until my doctor gave me a clue. That's how I got rid of my breast lumps. I fought the battle against excess estrogen and won. We have to realize this battle exists in the first place, in order to win it.

There are many factors that can cause estrogen to increase in the body. This increase causes the cells to replicate more frequently. For the sake of this book and to easily identify our battle against hormone caused, abnormal replication of cells, I am creating a term and referring to this enemy as *proestros*.

There are several ways to view the estrogen increase in our bodies. One is from the outside coming in. Another is from the insides not having balance from within. Either way you look at it, hormones, specifically estrogenic ones, are changing our bodies.

Some say these changes are due to increasing popularity of certain ways of living or cultural changes. These changes have been taking place since the 1960s. Examples of cultural changes are: more women not having children or putting off having children to later in life; increased used of hormonal birth control; patentable hormone supplementation; not breast feeding; increased abortions; and increase in stress i.e. women working and having children. Believe it or not, all of these factors change estrogens in the body due to the physical hormonally caused changes that take place in the breast. On an individual level, each cultural change shows an increased risk for breast cancer. These societal changes are creating biological changes within our bodies. Many of us have several of these factors going on just because of the times we live in!

Another, more significant way, that estrogen has increased in our bodies is with the increase in external and ingested estrogenic factors such as chemical, herbicide, pesticide and carcinogen use in the home. Pesticide and herbicide use had a major upswing 75 years ago and only started to go down slightly recently. Chemicals and pesticides mimic estrogens and go right into our body as imposters taking up the role of estrogen where they should not.

More and more chemical products are being produced that we utilize in our homes. The food storage and cooking tools as well as carpets and paints used in homes all have estrogenic compounds. The recent "going green" trend is lightening the burden of solvents and inhaled chemicals, but these chemicals are still popular and inside many products. Household products are factors we should be most concerned with because the estrogenic compounds are odorless and invisible.

Sugar also increases estrogen. Sugar consumption itself has significantly increased 30% over the last three decades. It is now commonplace for people to consume drinks with sugar on a daily basis.

In addition to these cultural and external changes, some of us do or will have normal changes that occur internally that affect hormones. These include an inability to process and break down estrogens and decreased production of progesterone after menopause. If we combine these normal processes with cultural, ingested and external sources of estrogen, then we end up with what we have today...estrogen overload.

An Array of Estrogenic Definitions

I am not the only one who notices there is a fight against estrogen. The drugs that are prescribed for many breast cancer patients, as mentioned earlier in this book, are described as ***anti-estrogens***. Anti-estrogens are substances (typically drugs) that block the production of estrogen or inhibit their effects. This term itself illustrates there is a battle against estrogen in our bodies.

Estrogen dominance

Estrogen dominance is a term coined by Dr. John R. Lee, M.D in his first book on natural progesterone entitled, *Natural Progesterone: The Multiple Roles of a Remarkable Hormone.* Estrogen dominance means there is a higher amount of estrogen compared to progesterone, which causes a number of unnatural symptoms.

A primary role of estrogen is to control the growth and function of the uterus. A majority of estrogens promote cell growth, primarily of the tissues responsible for reproduction. It is estrogen's ability to promote cell growth, that makes its excess such a dangerous promoter of cancer. There are several estrogens in the body. Two of the main estrogens that are known to control growth are estradiol and estrone. Patentable, synthetic progestins can perform the same functions as some human estrogens.

Estrogen dominance can be caused by the use of patentable hormones being utilized for birth control or menopause relief, and our exposure to pesticides, metalloestrogens, plastics, chemicals, industrial waste products, car exhaust, meat, body products and much of the carpeting, furniture and paneling that we live with indoors every day. Estrogen dominance may also be the lack of progesterone, which can happen naturally as hormones get out of balance as we age. In his book, *What Your Doctor May Not Tell You About Breast Cancer*, Dr. John R. Lee, M.D. wrote that progesterone can keep cancer-causing forms of estrogens in check. He also knew that weaker forms of estrogen, such as estriol, do not seem to promote cancer-causing cell growth and could actually help protect against breast cancer.

Dr. John R. Lee, M.D. believed that estrogen dominance is at the very heart of what promotes breast cancer. His term, estrogen dominance, was pivotal in bringing attention to our internal battle against estrogen.

Some of the estrogen dominance symptoms I had were: allergies, rashes, sinus congestion, breast tenderness, cold hands and feet, thyroid dysfunction, decreased sex drive, copper excess and zinc deficiency, fat gain, especially around the hips and thighs, fatigue, fibrocystic breasts, headaches, hypoglycemia, irregular menstrual periods, insomnia, magnesium deficiency, PMS and sluggish metabolism. That was a lot of symptoms! Things may not look so good if we don't get rid of this excess estrogen in our bodies. You can see which ones may be affecting you from the following list:

Estrogen Dominance Symptoms

The symptoms and conditions associated with estrogen dominance are:
Acceleration of the aging process
Allergies, including asthma, hives, rashes, sinus congestion
Autoimmune disorders such as lupus erythematosis and thyroiditis, and possibly Sjoegren's disease
Breast cancer
Breast tenderness
Cervical dysplasia
Cold hands and feet as a symptom of thyroid dysfunction
Copper excess
Decreased sex drive
Depression with anxiety or agitation
Dry eyes
Early onset of menstruation
Endometrial (uterine) cancer
Fat gain, especially around the abdomen, hips and thighs
Fatigue
Fibrocystic breasts
Foggy thinking
Gallbladder disease

Hair Loss
Headaches
Hypoglycemia
Increased blood clotting (increasing risk of strokes)
Infertility
Irregular menstrual periods
Irritability
Insomnia
Magnesium deficiency
Memory loss
Mood swings
Osteoporosis
Polycystic ovaries
Premenopausal bone loss
PMS
Prostate cancer (men only)
Sluggish metabolism
Thyroid dysfunction mimicking hypothyroidism
Uterine cancer
Uterine fibroids
Water retention, bloating
Zinc deficiency

Reprinted by permission of The Official Website of John R. Lee, M.D. –
www.JohnLeeMD.com

Xenoestrogens

There is another term that refers to the fight against estrogens.
Xenogenous is a term used for hormones that are produced outside the
body. Another variant of that, *xenoestrogen*, refers to synthetic or
natural chemicals that act like estrogens. Synthetic xenoestrogens are
compounds used in industry to manufacture items such as containers
or electrical components. These compounds include PCBs
(polychlorinated biphenyls), BPA (bisphenol-A) and phthalates. These
compounds have estrogenic effects on living organisms even though

they differ chemically from the estrogenic substances produced by the organism's internal naturally produced endocrine system.

Natural xenoestrogens are plant-derived and include phytoestrogens (plant estrogens) and fungi. Because the primary route of exposure to plant compounds is by consumption of phytoestrogenic plants, they are sometimes called "dietary estrogens". Mycoestrogens which are estrogenic substances from fungi, are another type of xenoestrogen that is inhaled.

This term illustrates there is a battle against the onslaught of hormone-like estrogen from outside our body. The term xenoestrogen is limiting to our battle against excess estrogen in that it does not include other external sources of estrogens such as pesticides or the actual internal specific estrogens themselves that promote cell growth.

Mitogen

Yet still, there is another term used by scientists to describe breast cancer growth promoters. The term is *mitogen*. This is a chemical substance that does not damage DNA but stimulates a cell to multiply. Patentable hormones fall under this category. These "gen" terms might be making you dizzy by now! Again, this term is limiting in that it only refers to cell promoters and does not include internal sources, external chemical sources or natural sources that also cause DNA or changes.

Endocrine Disrupting Compounds (EDCs)

Not to worry, there is yet another term called *Endocrine Disrupting Compounds (EDCs)*. The EPA has defined this as "an exogenous agent that interferes with synthesis, secretion, transport, metabolism, binding action or elimination of natural blood-borne hormones that are present in the body and are responsible for homeostasis, reproduction, and the developmental process."

The Endocrine Society has explained EDCs from a physiological perspective further to say that *"an endocrine-disrupting substance is a compound, either natural or synthetic, which through environmental or inappropriate developmental exposures, alters the hormonal and homeostatic systems that enable the organism to communicate with and respond to its environment."*

These compounds are typically your PCBs, dioxins, plastics like BPA, chlororganic pesticides like DDT, fungicides and pharmaceutical agents like DES. This term further expands the estrogenic realm that exists in our environment to include natural and synthetic but is still limiting in its definition. Even though EDCs make a case for environmental influences to our bodies, they still do not include the very thing inside our bodies that causes breast cancer cells to grow...the specific estrogens themselves like estradiol that increase cell growth along with other internal factors such as stress and external factors such as radiation.

There is a reason there are all these terms in existence. We are being barraged by hormones! And these terms keep expanding to include more and more estrogen sources! These terms imply that many processes of the hormonal system may be disrupted. However, the effect which we are most concerned with, is the process that causes tumor cells to grow. I found it interesting that dictionaries have a definition for an *antiestrogen* but none for *proestrogen*. This is why I came to the conclusion we need a new word, *proestro*, to encompass all sources and their contributing effect of tumor cell growth.

Proestro

A proestro is any animal or plant hormone in excess, synthetic hormone, food, metabolite of estrogen, stressor or any chemical or natural environmental substance that imitates or disrupts the estrogen cellular pathway thereby increasing cell growth and promoting tumor growth. Proestros disrupt the underlying cellular pathways that estrogen controls or maintains by changing enzyme bonds, damaging

DNA, clogging receptor sites, generating free radicals and degrading cell energy and structural components. The terms xenoestrogen, mitogen, endocrine disrupting compound and metalloestrogen describe various subsets of proestros.

Notice that proestros are not limited to breast cancer. They can also cause other hormonally induced cancers such as ovarian, cervical, prostate and thyroid cancers. For the purpose of this book, I am focusing research on breast cancer only.

It is no wonder that the answer to breast cancer keeps eluding us. Scientists try to isolate out what the "one thing" is that causes breast cancer, but they don't or can't often study all these proestros at once. However, there have been a few case control studies that tested the combined effect of several proestros, which did show a positive correlation to breast cancer.[23] [24] [25]

On an individual level, many proestros are shown to have significant correlations to breast cancer in cellular, animal and human population studies.[26] For instance, in a Canadian case-control study, women working in automotive plastics and food canning facilities had higher rates of breast cancer from 376 to 470% odds ratio, respectively. [27]

As you can see with all these definitions, there is a growing awareness of estrogenic components in our environment, and changing culture

[23] Ibarluzea Jm et al. Aug 2004 *Cancer Causes Control* "Breast cancer risk and the combined effect of environmental estrogens".

[24] Bonefeld-Jorgensen EC et al. Oct 2011 *Environ Health* "Perfluorinated compounds are related to breast cancer risk in Greenlandic Inuit a case control study".

[25] Ghisari M et al. Mar 2014 *Environ Health* "Polymorphisms in phase I and phase II genes and breast cancer risk and relations to persistent organic pollutant exposure: a case-control study in Inuit women".

[26] Brody, JG and Rudel RA 2008 *Breast Diseases: A Year Book® Quarterly* "Environmental Pollutants and Breast Cancer: The Evidence from Animal and Human Studies".

[27] Brophy JT et al. Nov 2012 *Environ Health* "Breast cancer risk in relation to occupations with exposure to carcinogens and endocrine disruptors: A Canadian case-control study".

that is affecting our bodies. Whether chemical or compound, ingested, applied or inhaled or the actual hormones themselves, proestros promote the natural effects of estrogen by abnormal cell replication and hence breast cancer. The increase in environmental and chemical estrogens, along with societal changes, are the main contributors for estrogen increase in our bodies. Here is a table I put together with examples of external and internal proestros that have an affinity for breast cancer.

Breast Cancer Proestro Table

Patentable Hormones	Man-made	Naturally made	Ingested
Provera	Phthalates i.e. DEP, MEP	Estrone in excess	Sugar
Progestin birth control pills 10+ yrs. i.e. *Levonorgestrel*	Smoking	Estradiol in excess	Phthalates, phthalic acid,
Menopause treatment i.e. *Prempro*	Pesticides i.e. DDT and Atrazine	16 alpha OHE1 in excess	Alcohol
Fertility Drugs i.e. *Clomid*	Radiation	Cortisol in excess (stress)	Processed Soy
DES while pregnant 1940-1971	Polycyclic Aromatic Hydrocarbon (PAH)	Phytoestrogens in excess (plant estrogens)	PFC i.e. Teflon
Anabolic Steroids	Benzene	rBGH or rBST (cow hormones)	Bisphenols i.e. BPA
	PCB	Aluminum and copper in excess, Arsenic, Cadmium	
	Parabens	Androgen or testosterone in excess	

Birth Control Increase and Breast Cancer

Along with the increase in use of patentable hormones to alleviate menopausal symptoms mentioned in Chapter 1, a major cultural change has taken place in the realm of birth control. Since its FDA approval in 1960, hormonal birth control methods have been on the rise.

National Health Statistics Report October 18, 2012

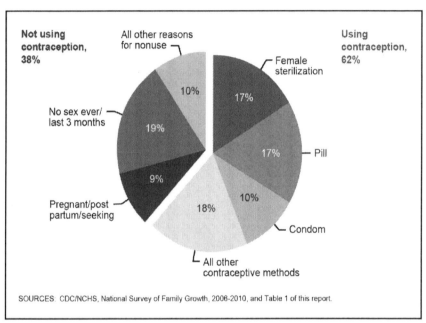

Figure 1. Percent distribution of women aged 15-44 years, by whether they are using contraception and by reasons for nonuse and methods used: United States, 2006-2010

In 1970, the safety of oral contraceptives was challenged and the formulation of the pill was changed. A year later, the Supreme Court legalized birth control for all citizens of the US, regardless of marital status. This opened up the door for all women to be able to utilize hormonal contraceptives.

As time went on, newer methods of birth control were made. The 1990s brought in the first contraceptive implant and the first injectable method ending with the first emergency contraceptive in 1999. In the 2000s the *Mirena*, a levonorgestrel releasing IUD, was introduced. In the same time period, the hormonal patch and the vaginal ring became available. In 2010, a new emergency contraceptive pill was released and shortly after that, in 2013, a new levonorgestrel releasing IUD (*Skyla*) was introduced. *Skyla* is smaller and has less hormone in it. Recently in 2013, the new Plan B emergency contraceptive pill became available without a prescription.

As you can see, the choices for women's hormonal birth control has increased over the past 50 years, as well as the availability for their use. According to the CDC, between 2006 and 2010, the birth control pill itself was used by 17% of women in the US. The oral contraceptive, or "pill" as it is known, has been shown to be helpful in many ways, but it has also been linked to breast cancer.

There has also been an increase in the number of women deciding to not have children in the US. This may be part of the reason for the increase in hormonal birth control use. The increase has gone from 10% in 1975 to 18% in 2000. When a woman decides not to have children, it affects a women's hormones in the breast cells leaving their breasts with a higher risk for breast cancer.

There are thousands of studies that have been done over the course of the pill's history, from its first formulations to the more recent lower dose formulations. A majority of these studies reflect an associated risk of breast cancer and there is no difference in which type of pill is taken, even though there are at least six different types of oral contraceptives, all with varying doses. In fact, secondary types of hormonal birth control, including the ring, patch, injectable and emergency contraceptive, also use the same patentable hormones as the pill. These other methods of hormonal contraception are not used as often, however. The IUD is the next most frequently used hormonal contraceptive (after the pill) at 2.4%.

For the purpose of reviewing hormonal contraceptives, I referred to studies performed on pill users. I found out there are two instances in a women's life where hormonal birth control is directly linked to breast cancer. One is when the pill is used before age 20, prior to pregnancy. The other is when the pill has been used for over eight years and the woman is currently or recently on the pill.

The Susan G. Komen website has posted a table of a pooled analysis of 54 studies of 53,297 women. It was published in 1996 and found between 20 to 104% increase in relative risk among women who were currently on the pill or who had been using the pill recently and had been using it for eight years or more.[28]

A study in 2014 showed a 45% increase in early onset of breast cancer for those women with a BRCA1 mutation and pill use prior to age 20.[29] So, here is an example of a recent study on current oral contraception that shows its effects. Should doctors be recommending gene testing for girls younger than age 20 prior to taking the pill? This amount of risk might be worth it! Or, maybe they could avoid it altogether and that would be a lot less expensive.

Looking at National Health Statistic Reports, I found that 16% of pill users use the pill prior to age 20. Combine the fact that most of these women utilize the pill over 10 years, this kind of birth control use significantly increases our risk to breast cancer. Luckily for us, that means that it is still safe to use after teenage years and for short periods of time. The only problem is, most of us stay on the pill for a majority of our lives.

There have been large studies that do not show a link between breast cancer and birth control at all, but I researched one of these studies and found that the actual control group was also taking birth control![30]

---

[28] Ww5.komen.org Susan G. Komen pooled analysis of 200 Breast Cancer Cases. *Table 9: Birth control pills and breast cancer risk.*

[29] Kotsopoulos J et al. Feb 2014 *Breast Cancer Res Treat* "Timing of oral contraceptive use and the risk of breast cancer in BRCA1 mutation carriers".

You would think the control group should not have been taking it! Additionally, in the progestin only group, they used only 31 cases (not large by any standard), which did find a 10% increase in risk. The length of the study was only four years and the ages of women were higher than other studies. The length of time of pill use was not analyzed. A significant amount of data was thrown out due to inconsistency or use of many formulations. The main purpose of the study was to determine if there was a difference in risk between formulations, not whether birth control caused breast cancer. As noted earlier, no difference in formulations was found. You can see how important it is to read studies!

Increase in Estrogenic Pesticides

As you can see from chapter one and column one in the proestros table, our cultural decision to use patentable hormones is not the only thing on the rise that induces estrogenic effects. Many pesticides and chemicals in use today also produce estrogenic effects on breast cells. Column two in the proestro table lists just some of these chemicals.

According to online databases (Mammary Carcinogens Review Database and Epidemiology Reviews Database) and a review volume titled "Environmental Factors in Breast Cancer" published by *Cancer* in 2008, at least 216 chemicals increased the number of breast cancer tumors in animal studies. Research has indicated that these common chemicals used in our environment cause breast cancer tumors, promote growth and even increase the cancer susceptibility in babies exposed to these chemicals in the womb.

When looking at the effects of pesticide and chemicals, scientists have been able to study the effect from many points of view. They include animal studies, human cellular studies and human population studies, all of which show the relevance of pesticides to breast cancer. So far,

---

[30] Marchbanks Polly A et al. April 2012 *Contraception* "Oral contraceptive formulation and risk of breast cancer".

cellular, animal and population studies have shown a 50 to 500% relative risk for women exposed to PCBs, DDT, PAH and chemical solvents.

Animal and human observational studies show the relevance of pesticides to breast cancer. Some chemicals such as DDT, atrazine and PCB (environmental contaminants that have been identified throughout the global ecosystem in fish, wildlife, and human tissue, including blood and breast milk) have shown the same effects as estrogen and can stimulate human breast cancer cells to grow.[31] One of the cellular studies in 1995 demonstrated that 16 alpha-OHE1 is raised due to atrazine, endosulfans, DDT and other pesticides.[32] 16 alpha-OHE1 is a human estrogen that in high amounts, is directly correlated with breast cancer growth, and is listed in column three of the proestros table.

There are several critical observational studies on humans that link breast cancer to pesticides.[33] [34] A population study in 2007 of young women exposed to DDT (an organochlorine), found a 500% increase in breast cancer risk.[35] A second 2010 human observational study in Poland linked breast cancer tumors directly to pesticides when breast cancer patients' tumor tissues had higher incidence of pesticides. Estrogenic tumors had a higher incidence of DDT, DDE, HCB and gamma HCH.[36] DDT, DDE, HCB and gamma HCH are all considered chloroorganic pesticides. Atrazine is also a chloroorganic pesticide that

---

[31] Smalling KL et al. Sep 2014 *Sci Total Environ* "Pesticide concentrations in frog tissue and wetland habitats in a landscape dominated by agriculture".

[32] Bradlow HL et al. 1995 *Environmental Health Perspective* "Effects of pesticides on the ratio of 16 alpha/2-hydroxyestrone"

[33] Westin Jerome B and Richter Elihu Nov 1990 Hebrew University "The Israeli Breast-Cancer Anomaly"

[34] Fenton SE *Endocrinology* 2006 "Endocrine-disrupting compounds and mammary gland development: early exposure and later life consequences".

[35] Cohn BA et al *Environmental Health Perspect* Oct 2007 "DDT and breast cancer in young women: new data on the significance of age at exposure".

[36] Ociepa-Zawal M et al. 2010 *J Environ Sci Health a Tox Hazard Subst Environ Eng* "Accumulation of environmental estrogens in adipose tissue of breast cancer patients".

has not been studied on humans and is the most widely used herbicide in the US. In animal studies, it has increased tumors in rats.[37] These chloroorganic pesticides store in our fat cells right there with our hormones.

A human study in 2004 on breast tissue revealed a similar correlation. Scientists measured 16 organochlorine pesticides and TEXB of 198 women at breast cancer diagnosis. They were compared to 260 women of matching ages without breast cancer. 40% of the study population had detected levels of the pesticides. There was an 84% correlation between aldrin and breast cancer and a 76% correlation between lindane and breast cancer among postmenopausal women.[38] As soon as these type of studies come out, the specific pesticide, such as DDT and lindane, gets restricted by the EPA. Regardless, many of these pesticides stay in our environment for a long time.

There are studies that do *not* show a link between pesticides and breast cancer. The problem I noticed with these studies, is that they typically test blood samples and not cell tissue. Pesticides are stored in tissue and are not as prevalent in the blood, except if recently exposed. In 2007, scientists performed a study researching the difference in taking blood (serum) versus tissue sampling. This study proved that estradiol is indeed stored in tissues involved in our endocrine system.[39] Scientists sampled tissues and took blood of women having cesareans and gynecological issues. Overall, there was a higher amount of free estradiol in tissue than in blood serum. Due to this, they recommended taking tissue samples for long term pesticide exposure analysis.

---

[37] Fukamachi K et al *Cancer Science* May 2004 "Possible enhancing effects of atrazine and nonylphenol on 7, 12-dimethylbenz[a]anthracene-induced mammary tumor development in human c-Ha-ras proto-oncogene transgenic rats".

[38] Ibarluzea, Jm, et al. Aug 2004 *Cancer Causes Control* "Breast cancer risk and the combined effect of environmental estrogens".

[39] Badeau M et al. Nov 2007 J *Clin Endocrinol Metab* "Estradiol fatty acid esters in adipose tissue and serum of pregnant and pre- and postmenopausal women".

Today, we can find studies where scientists are still taking serum samples. Since doing this type of sample will only give the current body pesticide burden, not all studies will show a correlation. Let's take a look at some graphs on the next two pages to further analyze this correlation. You can see that the pesticide use chart follows a similar line pattern as breast cancer incidence line graph from 1988 to 1998.

What the EPA pesticide graph does not show is the increase in pesticide use in earlier years. In 1960, 196 million pounds of herbicides/pesticides were used. In 1981 632 million pounds were used. That is an increase of 322%! It's a wonder that we think we can increase pesticides, by this much, with no human effects!

Pesticide Latency

The US Geological Survey states that there is a latency period for herbicides to get into the drinking water. It may take years, sometimes up to ten years. That still doesn't address inhaled pesticides or the ones we are actually eating. But as you can see, there is a resemblance in the direction these previous line graphs take. Pesticide and herbicides alike have increased over the past 83 years, especially from 1931 to 1961.

Latency: Tumor Start, Detection and Death

Unfortunately, incidence reports of breast cancer prior to 1975 are difficult to locate. Death rates are readily available which is why we find only death rate comparisons at earlier times. I did find some information that shows an increase in breast cancer incidence between the 1930s and 1978 by 40%. Another report states that breast cancer incidence increased by 53% between 1950 and 1989. Dr. Jonathan Wright states that from the mid-1940s to 1970s incidence climbed steadily and then in late 70s to early 80s the cancer rate began to accelerate by more than 300% with up to 200,000 new cases per year, 40,000 of them fatal.

The 80s also happens to be the time when women started using post-menopausal medications. During this time the rate for women under age 45 remained the same. Whatever the numbers and dates, we can see that breast cancer incidence has risen. According to the National Center for Health Statistics, there is a slight increase in breast cancer death rates from 1930 to 1947. This also happens to be the years where we see the sharpest increase in pesticide use. However, no breast cancer latency period would be taken into account in this example.

Breast cancer latency can be viewed as the time when a tumor cell starts to grow to when it becomes a detectable tumor. In many studies, there have been indicators of the actual time it takes for a tumor to form. One indication we have for tumor growth is from the WHI study when after five years, the study was halted due to women taking *Provera* for the duration of the study. Some of the tumors were detected within the first year! This was a very aggressive cancer. So, from this, we know it can take as little as one to five years in the case of aggressive exposure. Other studies linking radiation to breast cancer show it can take up to 35 years. A study by Dr. David Page on women who had abnormal breast cells, but not cancer, showed it took 14.8 years to appear.[40] However, the Breast Cancer Institute says that on average it

EPA Pesticides Data

Annual User Expenditures on Pesticides in the U.S.
By Pesticide Type, 1982 - 2007 Estimates
Agricultural Market Sector

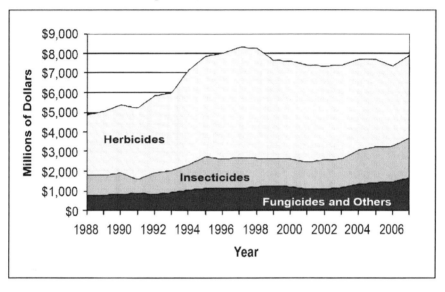

---

[40] Page DL, et al. Jan 2003 *Lancet* "Atypical lobular hyperplasia as a unilateral predictor of breast cancer risk: a retrospective cohort study".

Breast Cancer Incidence from 1975 to 2013 by SEER

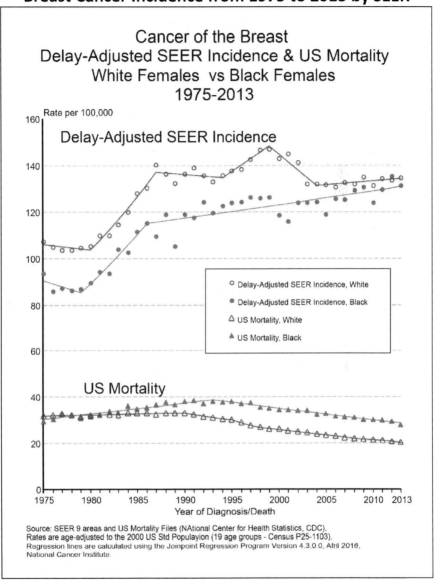

Cancer of the Breast
Delay-Adjusted SEER Incidence & US Mortality
White Females vs Black Females
1975-2013

Howlader N, Noone AM, Krapcho M, Miller D, Bishop K, Altekruse SF, Kosary CL, Yu M, Ruhl J, Tatalovich Z, Mariotto A, Lewis DR, Chen HS, Feuer EJ, Cronin KA (eds). SEER Cancer Statistics Review, 1975-2013, National Cancer Institute. Bethesda, MD, http://seer.cancer.gov/csr/1975_2013/, based on November 2015 SEER data submission, posted to the SEER web site, April 2016.

takes eight to ten years for a cancer cell to grow into a group of cells ½ inch in diameter. So, you can see that the time for a tumor to become detectable can vary based on the type of proestros, as well as, the quantity of proestros to which you have been exposed.

There are also indicators for breast cancer latency to be determined from tumor detection to death. An observational study took place on Israel in the 1980s. Westin and Richter noticed a sharp 8% decrease in breast cancer deaths ten years after DDT use was banned in Israel.[41] This may be an indicator of the latency period between high pesticide use and breast cancer death...ten years. This would be indicative of aggressive pesticide exposure along with a fast-growing tumor.

Between the 1930s and 1978, breast cancer incidence increased by 40%. Another report states that breast cancer incidence increased by 53% between 1950 and 1989. This increase happens to be at the same time as increased use of pesticides in the US.

Here is an observational correlation below. Based on the death latency discovered in the Israel study on DDT, I pulled maps ten years apart. Look at the map with breast cancer deaths from 2006 to 2010. Now look at the atrazine map from ten years earlier (1996). Atrazine is the most common herbicide used and found in our environment today. Isn't it weird that the mid-west states match up in both maps where atrazine, was sprayed? And this is a low estimate by the USGS of just one herbicide!

---

[41] Westin JB and Richter E Nov 1990 Unit for Environmental and Occupational Medicine "The Israeli Breast-Cancer Anomaly".

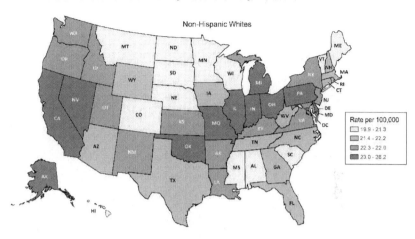

Map taken from www.cdc.gov

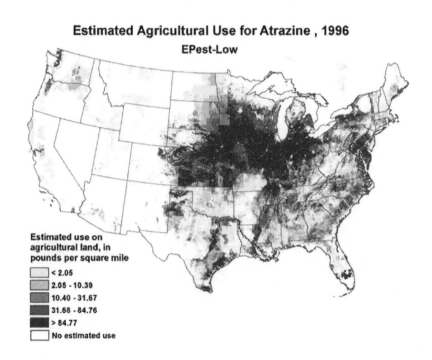

Map taken from http://water.usgs.gov website.

50

Then I wondered why the West coast had high death rates. Well, I looked it up, and in the West coast, paraquat (weed killer) and sermazine, two different herbicides are used. In a study in 2013, paraquat augmented cells with breast cancer BRCA1 defect.[42] Ok, so I don't want to get too excessive with maps, but here is your map of the West and East coast states with paraquat. How exciting.

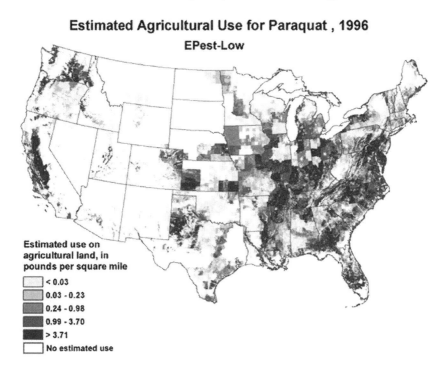

Map taken from http://water.usgs.gov website.

Now, these maps had me asking what about the states getting all these pesticides dumped on them from the Mississippi river, i.e. Mississippi. Oh, this is what happened to them. Take a look at the map showing African American breast cancer deaths. Of course! Mississippi has a higher African American population than average (37.4% for Mississippi). If you look at the numbers on each of the breast cancer

---

[42] Kang HJ et al. 2013 *J Toxicol Sci* "Correlations between BRCA1 defect and environmental factors in the risk of breast cancer".

maps, you can see that black women have a higher mortality rate, than white women. That is why there is such a disparity in these maps. Now this is just getting crazy!

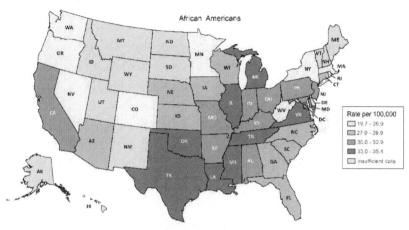

Map taken from www.cdc.gov

Now, I realize these correlations do not prove cause and effect, but they sure paint a picture for us. You can't help but notice the Northern states with small incidence, comparable with little pesticide use.

Not only can we visually see this strange correlation, but several of our own agencies believe the US is covered with pesticides that are affecting our health. Here is what they are saying:

Pesticides were found to exceed benchmarks in streams everywhere and increased by 90% from 2002 to 2011 in urban streams. 22% of wells exceeded benchmarks for pesticides in studies by the US Geological Survey published in 2014 and 2015. Pesticide residues have also been found in rain and groundwater.

The National Academy of Sciences estimates that between 4,000 and 20,000 cases of cancer are caused per year by pesticide residues in food in allowable amounts.

The United States Department of Agriculture and the United States Fish
and Wildlife Service estimate that between 6 and 14 million fish are
killed by pesticides each year in the US.

The Endocrine Society said this in a scientific statement in 2009:

*"In summary, exposure to estrogens throughout a woman's life,
including the period of intrauterine development, is a risk factor for the
development of breast cancer. The increased incidence of breast cancer
noted during the last 50 years may have been caused, in part, by
exposure of women to estrogen-mimicking chemicals that have been
released into the environment from industrial and commercial sources.
Epidemiological studies suggest that exposure to xenoestrogens such as
DES during fetal development, to DDT around puberty, and to a mixture
of xenoestrogens around menopause increases this risk. Animal studies
show that exposure in utero to the xenoestrogen BPA increases this
risk."*

Remember when bald eagles were listed as on the endangered species
list? Eagles have made a come-back! Well, scientists say that this is due
to the ban on DDT in the US. If they can make a come-back, so can we!

It may be easier to dismiss these observations as an overreach but it
doesn't go without saying that we should be careful about the amount
of pesticides we are allowing in our body, especially during pregnancy,
fetal development, infancy, puberty and menopause. Specifically, in
low amounts, pesticides have shown to cause all sorts of cancer. Some
pesticides and chemicals are lurking in places you never dreamed of!
Soon, I will uncover those places for you within the S.L.E.E.P. Method.

Now you see there are many ways estrogen is increasing in our society.
Two large contributors, as seen here, are patentable hormones and
pesticides. There are many more factors that include man-made
chemicals such as PCBs, smoking, PAHs and internal life factors that
increase estrogen. Those will be discussed in detail within the S.L.E.E.P.
Method. Each one is a proestro. Most of us have been affected by a few

or more of these factors! Next you will get to see how these proestros are affecting hereditary and HER2 types of breast cancer also.

Chapter 3

PROESTROS INFLUENCE OTHER CAUSES

You might be asking about the other 25% of breast cancer cases that are not hormonally induced, as I was. In fact, I wasn't even going to mention the other causes of cancer because I didn't think other causes were known or that these causes were influenced by proestros. Boy, was I wrong!

As I researched more, I was shocked to find that scientists have identified the reasons for most of the remaining types of breast cancers, too. The other types of breast cancers are caused by genetic defects, inflammation, enzyme imbalance and possibly bacteria and viruses. I also was surprised to find doctors who are treating breast cancer patients with these factors in mind. I was even more surprised to find that some of these defective gene types of cancer can have estrogenic and other hormonal influences!

As my mother said, while reading parts of this section, "this chapter is not for the lazy brain"! Here, we're going from the cellular level magnifying down to the DNA and gene level. Reading scientific information on genes takes concentration, so if you are tired or lack focus, you may want to move to skim over the details. However, this is the most interesting science that I found because many of us would not have guessed proestros influence these other causes.

Defective Genes

Yes, scientists have discovered other markers that cause breast tumor cells to replicate. They have found that breast cancer may be caused by tumor suppressor genes that have stopped functioning. These are called oncogenes to be exact. These oncogenes are the very genes that come along and find cancer defects in the genetics of cancer cells and then repair those defects and return them to a normal cell state. So these oncogenes get turned off and stop protecting against cancer. They can be inherited, or acquired then develop.

Before we go much further into defective oncogenes, it may be helpful to understand what a gene is. I will have to get a little more into technical science here, but hopefully defining gene will make the rest fairly easy to understand. Here is how a gene is defined:

A **gene** is the molecular unit of heredity of a living organism. It is used by the scientific community as a name given to some stretches of DNA (deoxyribonucleic acids) and RNA (ribonucleic acids) that code for a function in the organism. Living beings depend on genes. Genes hold the information to build and maintain an organism's cells and pass genetic traits to offspring. All organisms have genes corresponding to various biological traits, some of which are visible, such as eye color or number of limbs, and some of which are not, such as blood type, increased risk for specific diseases, or the thousands of biochemical processes that comprise life. The word *gene* is derived from the Greek word *genesis* meaning "birth", or *genos* meaning "origin"

HER2 Defective Gene

In breast cancer tumors, a few defective oncogenes were discovered in the 1970s. Scientists discovered oncogenes called HER2 (Human Epidermal Growth Factor Receptor 2), EGFR (Epidermal Growth Factor Receptor) and ras genes (an abbreviation for rat sarcoma). 15 to 20% of breast cancers test positive for the HER2 oncogene, which causes the genes to produce too much of the growth-promoting HER2 protein (neu protein).

HER2 is a type of EGFR gene that tells cells to grow. When there are too many copies of these genes, the grow message is increased. They create grow messages by producing neu growth-promoting proteins. Either the genes overabundance themselves, or the extra neu proteins can be found by testing. Tumors that test positive for HER2 tend to be more aggressive than estrogen positive tumors alone.

Patients who test positive for the HER2 oncogene can take a drug called Herceptin. Herceptin is a genetically engineered antibody that binds to the HER2 protein and was developed in 1991 with final clinical trials in 2003. In 1998, it was approved by the FDA.

HER2 proteins, called neu, are attached to HER2 genes within the cancer cell. These neu proteins are special in that they are the only ones that penetrate the cancer cell wall. By attaching to the proteins, Herceptin can enter the cell wall via the protein and block the HER2 growth factor receptor that causes the cancer cells to grow. In fact, it also shrinks the cancer tumors and some disappear completely.

Clinical trials in 1998 to 2003 demonstrated that Herceptin reduces the size of tumors in 25% of those with the HER2 gene. For those in late stage HER2 breast cancer, nearly half saw their tumors shrink, when combined with chemotherapy. For early stage cancer, HER2 patients had an increased survival rate of 33%.[43] This is a good example of medicine proving cancer tumors can shrink.

Herceptin would need to be taken long term as it stops recurrence of breast cancer in half after taking it for three years. Unfortunately, this drug comes with many side effects, including cardiac toxicity. This medication was a pinnacle of success for the medical industry and breast cancer because it triggered the first generation of modern drugs against cancer by targeting specific cancer genes that are over expressed.

Why does the body create extra copies of HER2 oncogene? The answer is actually found in studies. A study in 2013, showed that a *Substance P* and *NK-1R*, which are highly expressed in HER2 tumors, contribute to the increase of protein receptors in HER2 genes.[44] Okay, so if you are

---

[43] Porter Stanberry, publisher Oct 2014 "The Next Big Step Forward for Cancer Treatment".

like me, you may be wondering what the heck Substance P and NK-1R are. Well, it's a beyond the scope of this book, but they are considered neuropeptides and cytokines that are pro-inflammatory. This means they create inflammation. These inflammatory neuropeptides and cytokines attach to HER2 proteins and cause cell division.[45] They also cause resistance to HER2 drugs. So, in effect, HER2 is made due to inflammation.

In addition to its relationship to neuropeptide and cytokines, HER2 has been shown to be related to auto immune/inflammatory diseases such as Crohn's disease (inflammatory bowel)[46], and Hashimoto's (inflammatory thyroid)[47]. This tells us that auto immune response and inflammation of the body is related to, and an important factor in the way HER2 genes act. These are the reasons HER2 is known as *inflammatory breast cancer.*

Knowing this information is critical to help doctors realize that they can treat HER2 patients with natural inflammation reduction strategies, as well as whatever drugs are necessary. Treating inflammation in the body will help the breast cancer treatment drugs (Herceptin) be effective, as well as lower the risk of getting HER2 breast cancer again.[48] A simple C-reactive protein blood test can show levels of inflammatory markers.[49] After this, it can be ascertained where or why inflammation

[44] Garcia-Recio S et al. Nov 2013 *Cancer Res* "Substance P autocrine signaling contributes to persistent HER2 activation that drives malignant progression and drug resistance in breast cancer".

[45] Bhatelia K et al. Nov 2014 *Cell Signal* "TLRs" linking inflammation and breast cancer".

[46] Tsai MS, et al. Oct 2014 *Ann Surg Oncol* "Hospitalization for Inflammatory Bowel Disease is Associated with Increased Risk of Breast Cancer: A Nationwide Cohort Study of an Asian Population".

[47] Muller I et al. May 2011 *J Endocrinol Invest* "High prevalence of breast cancer in patients with benign thyroid diseases".

[48] Catania A et al. Aug 2013 *Breast Cancer Res Treat* "Immunoliposome encapsulation increases cytotoxic activity and selectivity of curcumin and resveratrol against HER2 overexpressing human breast cancer cells".

[49] Makboon K et al. Mar 2015 *Cancer Causes Control* Association between high-sensitivity C-reactive protein (hsCRP) and change in mammographic density over time

is showing up in the body and addressed accordingly. Identifying the cause of inflammation may not always be easy, but alternative and mainstream doctors are gaining a better understanding of inflammation in the body and from where it is derived.

I was surprised to see our friendly hormones showing up again, even with HER2. Patients who test positive for estrogen receptors and HER2 also have success with anti-estrogen drugs. 5 to 10% of tumors that test HER2 positive actually respond to estrogen blocking drugs.[50] The potential reason why anti-estrogenic drugs work, is that the breast tissue area surrounding these tumors is being strengthened by not allowing the cancerous cells out. Strengthening, in this case, means blocking estrogen in the remainder of the breast tissue and fat cells surrounding the tumor. How HER2 behaves is regulated by signaling through estrogen receptors. It is very possible that excess estrogen in the cell environment can help trigger the inflammatory response in HER2.

There's that estrogen again! Well folks, that brings the percentage of breast cancer being caused or influenced by excess estrogen up by about 1% for a total of 76%!

Pesticides and Gene Alteration

It is well known that genetic alterations are acquired versus being hereditary. It is also well known that hormones are carried by the blood and they regulate gene expression when entering cells. There is reason to believe the HER2, ras and/or EGFR genes have actually been modified by estrogen mimicking pesticides. There is evidence in amphibians and mammals that atrazine is an endocrine disrupter and can cause these gene changes.

---

in the SWAN mammographic density subcohort".
[50] Chakraborty AK et al Mar 2015 *Anticancer Res* "Co-targeting ER and HER family receptors induces apoptosis in HER2-normal or overexpressing breast cancer models".

In a study in 2005, scientists used rats with the same ras gene as humans. They showed that the Hras 128 was sensitive to getting breast cancer when given atrazine and nonylphenols. These herbicides caused genetic mutations early in the process of tumor development, prior to proliferation of cells and breast tumor creation.[51] The question is, will this same defect happen in humans?

The Breast Cancer Prevention Institute says that a metabolite of estrogen called 4-hydroxy-catecho estrogen quinone is found in higher levels of women with breast cancer. It is known to directly damage DNA.

Since it would be cruel to test humans with pesticides in order to monitor gene changes, experimental studies on humans will never occur. However, there have been several human cellular studies and many observational studies on humans and animals who have been exposed to pesticides.

On animals, scientists have studied the effects on fish, rats and amphibians. They have found that pesticides can cause defective ras genes, in addition to the hormonal changes I spoke of earlier. Scientists have ongoing studies on the effects on fish, amphibians and reptiles in wet locations and have found that atrazine, along with other pesticides, can cause defective genes at the concentrations that are found in the environment.

Based on observational studies, cellular experiments and scientific studies on animals, along with what some of our government agencies are saying, there are many people who believe there is a high probability that exposure to pesticides can alter the human gene and cell make-up and over time cause breast cancer and even death. There is also evidence that has demonstrated that exposures must be considered cumulatively because compounds accumulate over time.[52]

---

[51] Tsuda H et al. Jun 2005 *Cancer Science* "High susceptibility of human c-Ha-ras proto-oncogene transgenic rats to carcinogenesis: a cancer-prone animal model".

60

The way in which they can alter genes are two-fold. First, they can do so utilizing hormones. Secondly, they can cause changes utilizing enzymatic pathways.

These chemicals added to our daily exposure to stress, lack of sleep, viruses, carcinogens, smoking and pollution, all work together to silence cancer repair genes. Many of these do so by using estrogen. Hormones themselves are genetic switches. Estrogens specifically work to activate certain genes and de-activate others. What we can prove is that herbicides, pesticides and fungicides like atrazine are in our drinking water, soil and food; have affected fish, amphibian and reptile hormones, genes and reproductive systems; herbicide and pesticide use has increased over the past 85 years; and banned pesticides, as well as pesticides that are currently being utilized, show clear evidence of hormonal changes at the cellular level in both animals and humans.

Conservationists are trying to find ways to reduce pesticide load on animal species by land modifications. Who is going to help reduce our load? Where is our land modification? Well, as it turns out, scientists are also studying ways to remove these contaminants from our environment. They have developed a few types of filtration systems, but they are trying to improve their usability.

Inflammation, viruses or bacteria may have been what caused most genetic mutations in breast cancers prior to herbicide and patentable hormonal use. Although I found no specific virus or bacterial infection directly corresponding to breast cancer to date, there are many cancers that have been found to be caused by viruses and bacteria. We cannot rule them out as a possibility for the remaining breast cancers that are not linked to any specific cause.

---

[52] Kortenkamp A *Int J Androl* 2006 "Breast cancer, oestrogens and environmental pollutants: a re-evaluation from a mixture perspective".

Hereditary Breast Cancer Genes

Lastly, we have a remaining 5 to 10% of breast cancer which is considered hereditary. Basically, a family member passes on an altered gene. In some cases, the gene that is passed down may not be a known gene, but it is considered hereditary none the less. For example, perhaps a daughter inherited a gene to begin menarche (menstruation) at an early age. Early menarche is known to be an increased risk for breast cancer because the women is exposed to more estrogen throughout her life. This is an example of how hereditary breast cancer can also be estrogen related. Estrogen is what initiates menarche.

BRCA Defective Gene

There are a few genes that scientists have identified as hereditary. One of these is the BRCA gene (BRCA1 and BRCA2). Many people who do not test positive for estrogen, progesterone or HER2 gene (Triple Negative), will test positive for mutated BRCA1 gene. 90% of people having hereditary breast cancer will test positive for this mutated gene. However, only 6% of women with breast cancer have this mutated gene. This type of cancer is generally more aggressive and fast growing. The lifetime risk for developing breast cancer for people who test positive for BRCA gene is 50 to 80%.

It is important to understand these inherited gene cancers still had to have another factor in order for it to develop. Basically, they are just starting off with an already defective gene. All they need are some other factors in sequence to get it started. It may be the very factors I described previously or other ones such as radiation. That is why it is imperative that BRCA carriers are very careful about proestros! They should definitely consider doing the S.L.E.E.P. Method!

In fact, even though BRCA 1 cancers test estrogen-receptor negative, they have also been shown to be responsive to estrogen lowering drugs! Dr. Susan Love has explained that the surrounding cells of the

BRCA 1 gene might be responding to estrogen outside the cell and sending signals to the cancer stem cells.[53] This makes total sense!

Additionally, there is more reason to believe that external factors may have been the culprit in changing these genes in the patient originally. A human cellular study in 2002 showed that some organochlorines in our environment have the capability to alter the expression of the tumor suppressor gene BRCA1 and therefore breast cancer risk.[54] Also, scientific studies show that 80% of women who have the BRCA1 gene mutation have a basal type of cancer. Basal clusters indicate gene mutations are most likely *not* inherited. Even though BRCA is considered a hereditary gene and there are new drugs targeting repair of these genes, a Dr. Stanislaw Burzynski has found that his antineoplastons can work on BRCA genes to get their cancer protective capability turned back on.[55]

P53 and CHECK2 Defective Genes

Two other less common mutations associated with increased risk of breast cancer are tumor suppressor genes p53 and CHECK2. The p53 gene prevents mutated cells from dividing and replicating. In 1998 there was a cellular study that showed that regular old progesterone activates this cancer protective gene.[56] With this study, we can see first-hand how hormones can affect genes, with progesterone demonstrated as a protective hormone, in this case.

CHEK 2 defect is common in women of northern and eastern European decent. It doubles breast cancer risk, but also is estrogen positive. Here

---

[53] *Dr. Susan Love's Breast Book* by Dr. Susan Love Chapter 4 p 101-128
[54] Rattenborg T et al. 2002 *Breast Cancer Res* "Inhibition of E2-induced expression of BRCA1 by persistent organochlorines".
[55] *Knockout* by Suzanne Somers p 67-8
[56] B. Formby and T.S. Wiley Sansum Medical Research Foundation in Santa Barbara, CA, 1998 *Annals of Clinical and Laboratory Science* that estrogen added to breast cancer cell cultures activated the oncogene (cancer-causing gene) *bcl-2*, whereas progesterone activated the cancer-protective gene called *p53*.

is yet another example of how important it is to contain estrogen! The percentage just keeps rising! Scientists are busy finding markers, DNA changes and links, but the information is not being communicated and addressed at the patient level for most of the breast cancer population.

PALB2 Defective Gene

An article in *Reuters* in August 2014 has revealed another hereditary gene... the PALB2. Of the very few people who have PALB2 mutations, 35% have a risk of getting breast cancer by age 70.[57] Testing is available internationally for this mutated gene. There are drugs called PARP inhibitor drugs (i.e. Lynparza™ and Veliparib) that are showing success in clinical trials against breast and ovarian cancer caused by this mutation.

PARP (poly ADP ribose polymerase) is a backup DNA enzymatic repair system found in the nucleus of a cell. When over activated by damaging effects, PALB2 uses up its needed components for repair and may become inactivated. PARP enzymes rebuild the PALB2 repair genes so PALB2 can function again. This repair system is activated to repair damaged cells when there is DNA damage induced by metabolic, chemical or radiation exposure. Conversely, these new drugs are targeting this enzymatic pathway to *decrease* enzymes to have the opposite effect on the cancer cell. PARP inhibitors disable the tumor cell's ability to repair its damaged DNA with little or no effect to normal cells.

Surprisingly, PARP enzymes are also essential in repairing inflammatory genes, the main issue concerning HER2 mutations. Scientists are finding that PARP inhibitors are showing a positive effect on HER2 overexpression as well as PALB2.[58] [59]

---

[57] Kate Kelland *Reuters* Aug 2014 "Study finds a gene mutation increases breast cancer risk to 1 in 3".

[58] Garcia-Parra J, et al. Oct 2014 *Eur J Cancer* "Poly (ADP-ribose) polymerase inhibition enhances trastuzumab antitumour activity in HER2 overexpressing breast cancer".

Triple Negative Breast Cancer

Another interesting fact I found in a 2015 article is that Triple Negative Breast Cancer (TNBC) has a 25 to 75% chance of testing androgen positive.[60] Oh my goodness! Can you believe there may be another hormone involved with breast cancer? Well, androgens happen to be a precursor to estrone, one of the estrogens that increases cell growth. So, are you surprised?

It is believed that androgens play an important role in the synthesis of estrogen in adult women. Androgens also regulate a woman's body before, during and after menopause. Androgens, a precursor steroid to all estrogens, are stimulated by testosterone conjugates. Testosterone is the primary androgen and the principal male sex hormone, but is also produced in small amounts by women's ovaries and adrenals. If a women's testosterone and androgen levels are not proper, the whole body can be affected. Currently, clinical trials are being conducted for TNBC patients with a new androgen blocking drug. It is important to note that there are ways to regulate these hormones using natural methods without side effects.

You can see why it is important for you to find out your hormonal levels as early as possible. It is equally important to balance out your hormones by getting proestros out of your life. Not only is it important for your own health, but it is important for your offspring's health so they don't receive your defective oncogenes!

[59] Nowsheen S et al. Sep 2012 *Cancer Res* "HER2 overexpression renders human breast cancers sensitive to PARP inhibition independently of any defect in homologous recombination DNA repair".
[60] Safarpour D and Tavassoli FA May 2015 *Arch Pathol Lab Med* "A targetable androgen receptor-positive breast cancer subtype hidden among the triple-negative cancers".

Chapter 4

GET THE PROESTROS OUT OF HERE!

Summing Up the Cause

To sum it all up, breast cancer is caused by increasing cell production of cancer cells. Most of the time this happens due to proestros acting on estrogen or estrogens themselves acting alone. But proestros can also alter genes and reduce needed enzymes in the body. As mentioned before, proestros are not the only thing that can cause gene and enzyme modifications. Inflammation and imbalance of enzymes can too, but proestros are a very, very large part of these gene changes.

Here is the breast cancer breakdown. Up to 75% of breast cancer tests estrogen/progesterone positive, or in other words is caused by excess estrogen. 20 to 25% is caused by extra copies of the HER2 oncogene. HER2 expression is found to be due to inflammation. 5 to 10% of HER2 is also influenced by excess estrogen surrounding the tumor (1% of all breast cancers). Up to 10% is triple negative or hereditary including BRCA1, BRCA2, PALB2, p53, CHECK2 gene defects. 25 to 75% test positive for androgens or may be caused by proestros. 2 to 5% of breast cancer is known to be from radiation. But, radiation is also linked to an increase in estrone and testosterone. That brings us to a total of 78 to 89% or more of breast cancer being caused or influenced by proestros!

Since there are so many sources of excess estrogen, I have created a table in Part II where you can see where your highest risks lie. External proestros and sugar all have increased estrogenic tendencies and have the highest relative risks associated with breast cancer.

Controlling Proestros

The best prevention therefore, is eliminating all or most known potential compounds and triggers (proestros) that increase estrogen. If you have already been exposed to chemicals and pesticides, it is critical to get these out of the body. In order to do this, we can take several steps as I have outlined in the S.L.E.E.P. method in Part III of this book. I know I'm saving all the good stuff for the end. Even if you decide to do only some of the S.L.E.E.P. methodology, you can significantly decrease your breast cancer risk.

You see, sometimes prevention ends up being the cure for the population as a whole. Before seat belts were required in cars, there were money making machines for brain injuries. There were all sorts of equipment being made to cure people who had injuries from accidents. Once seat belts came into existence and caught on, the brain injury money making machine died out.

Fast forward to today and the same thing is happening. The medical industry is making its money on mammogram machines, surgeries, chemo and drugs. Pharmaceutical companies are trying to make a pill or anti-estrogen patch. Pharmaceutical, chemo and mammogram corporations send their representatives with their products to the FDA and National Cancer Institute in order to get product approval. These companies are the prime sources who are trying to help us find a cure after breast cancer has occurred. However, pharmaceutical companies have not been successful making any anti-estrogens without severe side effects and none have been FDA approved to prevent breast cancer before it starts.

Low income producing methods such as supplements; vitamins or herbals are lost because most of these manufacturing companies do not have the money to get their products through the FDA process. Additionally, many supplements are not high quality and do not have the same effectiveness as high quality supplements. Until people cause a change in market demand, the medical industry will continue to be the primary source at work for us.

Other medical issues and other hormonal factors can play important roles in healing because our body works together in one system. Not one formula is right for every individual. Hormonal and genetic triggers such as bacterial infections, viruses, improper gut flora, mold, inflammation and others can influence your healing. I would love to talk more about those too, but will have to save my enthusiasm for other books. You may need to re-visit these issues if you are having trouble healing.

The focus of this book is on reducing your proestro load, getting out excess estrogen and hormone balancing; the direct items that most influence breast cancer growth. It would be nice to think that prevention for breast cancer is easy and quick, but it is a slow process.

Our society is at a crossroads. We work hard at home and our jobs. We don't have the time to look into our food products, the very things we are putting on our body or to research alternative medical technology. It is so much easier to just buy what is packaged for us at the grocery store or do what the doctors say to do. But a few minutes extra at the store or online, can be a life changer. Taking an active part in our health versus being reactive can make a difference. It is my hope that through increasing awareness of proestros and utilizing these methods, our society can reduce breast cancer causes by 75% or more!

What proestros can you control? Well it's good to know that you actually can control most of them to a certain extent. It depends on your commitment and discipline of course.

Hormone Filter

First, we need to understand a little about the hormonal system in our body. Dr. John R. Lee, M.D systematically and scientifically breaks down the how and why hormones work in the body. Some parts are tedious to read because it is so much medical detail... unless you are into that sort of thing. I just want to make it easy for you so here I go with a couple of Dr. Lee's main ideas.

The most important thing to realize is there is *no* filter for hormones that are put on your skin. Hormones that are taken in through the skin are absorbed *directly* into your body's cells. For example, doctors prescribe "the patch" for birth control or hormone replacement therapy. The patch is meant to deliver a slow dose of synthetic estrogen, estradiol or progestin in your body, through the skin. Anything you put on your skin (from the patch to lotion) or put in your uterus is absorbed and stored directly in the fat cells.

Unfortunately, most hormones are ingested. You may be taking a birth control pill right now. The food you eat may have hormones in it or the containers you use may have xenoestrogens in them. There are filters for ingested hormones. They are your kidneys and liver. They filter hormones like they filter food. Most natural and bioidentical hormones will process through and are excreted through the urine. So any "natural to your body" hormones will process through the kidneys and urine. Any extraneous synthetic, patentable or unnatural hormones process through the small intestine wall and accumulate in the liver overtime. These extraneous proestros are not good for the body.

Other Sources of Proestros

Our body treats a lot of things like estrogen, even when they are not. Some things we intake through our mouths create higher estrogen levels or mock estrogen in our bodies. As discussed earlier, the term xenoestrogens has been coined for this effect. Most of these categories are listed in the proestros table under foods and chemicals. Proestros come in Teflon pans, plastic water bottles, and in plastic food storage. Remember the big scare of bisphenol-A, otherwise known as BPA, in plastic water bottles? Yes, they emit estrogen like particles - xenoestrogens. We were letting our babies drink from baby bottles made out of this stuff! We were taking water bottles to the gym and leaving them in a car so they can bake some delicious xenoestrogens.

Other things we ingest are in our foods. Foods these days come with yummy chemicals and growth hormones that we can't even taste. Cosmetics that we apply to our skin like lotions, deodorant and cosmetics have estrogen mocking chemicals that go directly into our blood stream or cells through our skin. But, it is likely that the largest contributors of proestros throughout our modern life are pesticides and external chemicals and metals.

Wherever we have gotten high amounts of xenoestrogens, synthetic estrogen, extra estrogens throughout our life, it builds up in the body. Your body stores the excess hormones in the part of the body with the most amount of fat cells, the breast tissue. In the next section, you will get to find out if you have these excess hormones in your body.

Can you control proestros? The real questions are:
Can you control what birth control you use?
Can you control what you eat?
Can you control what you use to cook and store food?
Can you control what products you put on your body?
Can you control stress in your life?

Like *Bob the Builder* says … Can we do it? YES, WE CAN!

PART II

HORMONE TESTING AND PLANNING

Chapter 5

SOME LUMP IN BETWEEN

Checking for Lumps: What's normal?

We all know that we have to watch out for lumps. We are told to feel around for extra bumps or lumps that are getting bigger. That's how most women find out they have breast cancer. However, for some of us it is difficult to tell the difference between an unusual lump and a normal lump. Most of us are some lump in between small lumps, lots-o-lumps or large lumps. How are we supposed to keep track of these lumps? Why are we so lumpy and is this normal? Do we have a greater risk of breast cancer with more lumps?

To understand the lumpy parts of our breasts we need to understand breast anatomy. Breasts are mostly made up of fat cells and connective tissues including lymph vessels and milk lobes. Our breasts develop during puberty. Part of that development involves the milk duct lobules and ducts. The lobules are what make milk during lactation. Milk is generated from the lobules, passes into the ducts and out several openings in the nipple. How these lobules grow and mature can affect breast cancer risk.

A lobule is a milk duct with surrounding ductules which are the glands that make milk. When you are born, you have *Type 1* lobules. 85% of breast cancer grows in Type 1 milk duct lobules. At puberty some of these Type 1 lobules develop into Type 2 lobules. Type 2 lobules are where 15% of all breast cancer starts. By the end of puberty, you end up with 75% Type 1 and 25% Type 2 lobules. If you become pregnant, the breasts grow and double in volume by producing more Type 1 and 2 lobules. By the middle of the second trimester, 70% of the breast lobules become another type: Type 4. At full term 85% are Type 4. After pregnancy, they revert to Type 3. Both Type 3 and Type 4 lobules are resistant to cancer because their cells copy their DNA slowly. After menopause, 20% of women have their lobules retire completely, which is referred to as involution. Women whose lobules that have gone through involution, have a significantly decreased risk of breast cancer.

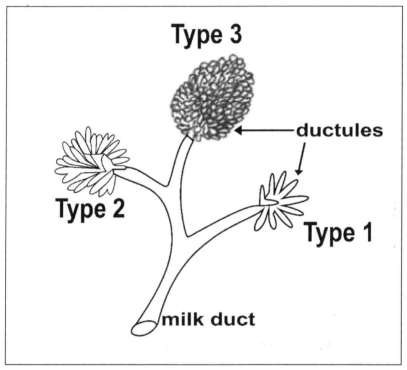

Schematic of breast lobules

Diagram printed with permission from www.bcpinstitute.com

Breasts have fatty tissue that grows around the milk ducts. For most of us, this fat results in a bumpy uneven surface. If you feel like your breasts are similar to bubble wrap or gravel on a driveway, don't panic! These are normal lumps. There is also a ridge of fat that develops at the bottom of the breast called the infra-mammary ridge. This is also a natural source of uneven texture.

Along with fat, non-cancerous, normal variations or *original* lumps will appear grey on a mammogram. The more fat there is, the greyer the mammogram will be. Denser areas will show up lighter or white. The lighter areas are the fibrous, connective and glandular tissues, including milk ducts and lymph. These fibrous and glandular tissues make up the density of a breast. As you will see later on, high breast density, especially after age 50, is correlated with increased risk of breast cancer. Milk ducts and lymph are the areas where breast cancer typically grows. As mentioned earlier, 85% of all breast cancers start in the milk ducts.

Other developments that occur in the breast are the lymph glands and vessels. These lymph vessels collect debris from cells and strain it through lymph nodes and then back into the blood stream. This lymphatic system helps fight infection. It is your breast cleaning station. In fact, when your body is sending out the cancer cells or dead cells, they have to go back somewhere. They go into the blood stream and ultimately into the lymph filter, kidney or liver.

Dominant Lumps

The thing you are noticing or looking out for when you do a self-exam is a dominant or unusual lump. These are lumps that have grown in your breast after puberty. Lots of times, breast changes occur in our 30s and 40s prior to menopause and then again after menopause. There is no medical consensus as to why this happens, but these are the years when you are most likely to find an unusual lump. These types of lumps are not always cancerous, but when they do turn out to be cancerous and are growing in the ducts or lobules, they are typically found to be estrogen positive tumors.

You may notice, if you are pre-menopausal, that your *original* lumps are swollen and sore when you are mid-cycle or right before your period. Scientists know this happens due to hormonal changes in the body. This is called *cyclical pain*. What is amazing to me is that to this day, they don't know why this happens. They don't know the exact pathways, if you will. So far, there seems to be a lot of questions about how the breast interacts with the body.

Breast Functionality

Well I don't know about you, but I can tell that cyclical hormones make the breast swell especially in certain areas of the lymph vessels. The swelling presses on the surrounding nerves and voila, you have some pain! Scientists have treated women's breast pain effectively with hormonal blocking drugs. Do you think maybe hormones are at the root cause of the pain? This kind of stuff is just weird to me. You mean to tell me, scientists have been studying breasts for years, searching for a breast cancer cure and they don't even know how the breast works???

Isn't it common sense that if your car breaks down, the mechanic can fix it because he understands how it works? If your house has a plumbing leak, the plumber has to know how plumbing works in order to fix it. Why then, would they spend countless hours taking samples of breast and cancer tissue under the microscope, adding this or that to see the reactions, but not study mammalians to understand how this very important integral part works; the pathways, the t-cells, the genetics, the lymph, the milk ducts, the fat. How do all these interconnect?

Thank goodness for doctors who are doing research on how the body works. A retired breast cancer surgeon, Dr. Susan Love, has studied milk ducts and lobes and has found that they work together with the surrounding fatty tissue in a sort of community. The fat and the milk ducts may actually exchange hormones and information.[61] Who would have thought my fat was talking to my hormones?

Breast cancer cells can exist in our bodies without growing or causing harm. A study by Mina Bissell, a researcher in Berkeley, CA, showed that nests of tumor cells were lying dormant in 39% of breasts.[62]

---

[61] *Dr. Susan Love's Breast Book* by Susan M. Love, MD 2010 p 121-124

Scientists have also found that those cancer cells will not grow unless they are in the right environment. Dr. Bissell studied the environment surrounding breast cancer cells in breast tissue and found that cancer cells can act like normal cells if they are in a normal breast environment. They will behave so to speak. This explains why tumors can appear to be dormant or sleeping for years and then a patient can have a recurrence. If we know what the environment is doing, we can keep those breast cancer cells asleep permanently! We don't have to know the exact pathways and intricacies to get a really good picture of what causes breast cancer.

Other Lumps

Lumps can be fibrous, called fibroadenomas. These are simply cells that have over replicated in the milk lobules, fueled by estrogen. These types of lumps feel hard, smooth and round. Lumps can also be fluid filled sacs called cysts. These typically grow in women when they are in their 30s, 40s or 50s. Surface cysts feel like cysts, which are soft. Deeper cysts can feel harder due to layers of tissue and may be more difficult to differentiate.

Both of these lumps are related to hormonal changes and are considered normal. But are they? How do we know the difference between cells that have over replicated for no apparent reason and ones that are cancerous? Fibroadenomas can be aspirated or biopsied to verify what they are. They typically develop right after puberty and never turn into breast cancer. Cysts can be aspirated to remove the fluid if they are painful. They are not linked to a higher risk of cancer either, so these two types of lumps are normal.

---

[62] Tonnov-Jessen L, Bissell MJ Jan 2009 *Trends Mol Med* "Breast cancer by proxy: can the microenvironment be both the cause and consequence?"

Inflammation

It is well known that our body responds to bacterial and viral infections by inflammation of the nasal passages; direct blows by swelling around the affected area; and common sense tells us that pre-menstruation causes swelling of the breasts. Inflammation is so much a part of our body, but it is treated as if it is an isolated event. In fact, inflammation is a visible sign that the body is in distress in various parts. But certain parts of the body or the entire system can become inflamed without us realizing it.

There are many factors that can cause inflammation and I won't go into all of them here. Basically, inflammation is a reaction in the body against a harmful stimulus. The main things we need to watch for are: foods that we are allergic or sensitive to, the lack of nutrients or too many of certain nutrients. It is important to have a balanced diet. Just because you are eating mountains of spinach or kale, doesn't mean it's balanced. Too much spinach can be difficult to digest and cause inflammation.

Blood tests can determine a patient's inflammation levels. High inflammation levels are associated with breast cancer patient's reduced survival time. A new study in March 2015 illustrates that inflammation may prevent breast density from decreasing as we age. A blood test marker for inflammation called C-reactive protein, if high, is associated with this slower decline in breast density.[63]

The body reacts to breast cancer the same way it does to a direct blow. Inflammation surrounds the cancer in response to its growth. What is not well known is that estrogen can increase or decrease inflammation based on the environment. Any increase in proestros can trigger estrogen which then triggers inflammation. The inflammation itself can

---

[63] Makboon K et al. Mar 2015 *Cancer Causes Control* "Association between high-sensitivity C-reactive protein (hsCRP) and change in mammographic density over time in the SWAN mammographic density subcohort."

become an environment that is conducive to cancer growth, including breast cancer. This is why in part of the S.L.E.E.P. Method we will be working on reducing inflammation, along with proestro reduction.

Breast Density

Breast density is used to describe how breasts look on a mammogram. It's not something describing how your breasts feel. A mammogram compares the fatty gray areas to the white lymph, ducts and lobules areas. Having high breast density means that you have more white areas than gray. Low breast density means that you have more fat and grey areas. Unfortunately, there is no exact science at this time for measuring density and it is not used by doctors to assess risk.

Increased breast density is directly linked to breast cancer. [64] [65] Women with high breast density are four to five times more likely to get breast cancer than women with low density.[66] In fact, it is not only linked, there are studies showing density directly correlates with a higher percentage of malignant type tumors and estrogen positive tumors.[67]

Realizing that breast density has a strong correlation with breast cancer, scientists are finding ways to decrease density utilizing drugs. Scientists have performed trials with drugs such as *Metformin* to decrease breast density. A Russian study in 2012 showed *Metformin* can reduce breast density around 28% of the time.[68] This drug is used to decrease glucose production from the liver. I bet you can guess what glucose does to estrogen. You'll find out more about it in the first "E"

---

[64] Ahmadineajad N et al. Dec 15 2013 *Iran Red Crescent Med Journal* "Association of mammographic density with pathologic findings".

[65] Boyd NF et al. Jan 18 2007 *N Engl J Med* "Mammographic density and the risk and detection of breast cancer".

[66] Ww5.komen.org/BreastCancer/HighBreastDensityonMammogram.html

[67] Keller BM et al. Mar 27 2014 *Proc SPIE* "Breast density and parenchymal texture measures as a potential risk factors for Estrogen-Receptor positive breast cancer".

[68] Bershtein LM et al. 2012 *Vopr Onkol* "The influence of metformin and N-acetylcysteine on mammographic density in postmenopausal women".

section of the S.L.E.E.P. method. Tamoxifen reduces density almost immediately. Doesn't it sound like estrogen has something to do with increasing density? Why shouldn't decreasing density be part of our health goals?

Even though there are conflicting measurement tools and beliefs about density, we can have some control over it. It may seem to make sense then, that if we could lower our breast density on our own, then we would have less risk of breast cancer. Synthetic menopausal hormone therapy is known to increase density as soon as you start taking it. You can certainly stop taking it to decrease density!

It takes a while for cancerous lumps to develop in the body. Our body grows fibrous or scar like tissue around cancerous lumps as they get larger. The body doesn't react to cancer when it is tiny. When breast cancer is detected, the lump is typically over one centimeter. If abnormal or dominant lumps in your breast are not kept under control, they can turn into abnormal cells and evolve into cancer. But good for us, we CAN keep our lumps under control. It has been proven thousands of times. I did it myself! Even cancer cells can be guided back to a normal growth pattern without using drugs or surgery.[69] Not all cancer can be detected as lumps, but even if they are just sitting there unbeknownst to you, you can shrink them!

Typically, a woman's breast density decreases after menopause because estrogen production goes down. Even though estrogen production decreases, this doesn't mean that breast cancer risk is reduced after menopause. In fact, risk of breast cancer goes up. For women whose breast density does not decrease as they age, there is an even higher risk for breast cancer. Obese women also have a higher risk because as they age, they have more fatty tissues.

---

[69] Sherry Baker from Health Sciences Jan 2, 2013 "Proof: Breast cancer cells can revert to normal without drugs".

Breasts are the accumulation of life. If you had cysts and replicated cells before menopause, they don't just go away. You have to make them go away. That is exactly what we are doing in the S.L.E.E.P. Method. Within this method, you will see how you can manipulate lymph, to keep proestros away from your ducts and lobes, where the majority of cancers start.

Fat Cells, Estrogen and Breast Cancer

The older you get; the higher risk of breast cancer you have. Breast cancer can occur in your 30s and 40s but there is a much higher incidence after age 50 (80% of all breast cancer occurs after age 50). The reason for this increase in risk is, that estrogens have accumulated and stored in your fat cells over time. Endocrine disrupters (proestros) tend to have a high solubility (dissolve easily) in lipids (fat) but not in water. That is why they accumulate in fat cells. Most fat cells are in the breast, thighs and abdomen. The breast ends up being a place with a high amount of proestros and estrogens. According to a study in 2006 by Yager and Davidson, estrogen levels are 10 to 50 times higher in breast tissue than in blood.[70]

Estrogen is stored in your fat cells over time, but did you know that fat cells also manufacture a small amount of estrogen themselves? The breast tissue has an enzyme called aromatase, which converts testosterone and androstenedrine into estrogen. When the body stops producing estrogen and progesterone on its own, the aromatase becomes more active and your body begins to move fat to the belly.[71] This creates an imbalance in hormones after menopause. Estrogen that was built up in the breast fat cells may remain and be higher after menopause due to this change. Since progesterone is no longer being made by the body, the estrogen does not have protective progesterone

---

[70] Yager and Davidson 2006 *New England Journal of Medicine Review* "Estrogen Carcinogenesis in Breast Cancer"

[71] Santosa S of Concordia University and Jensen M D of Mayo Clinic *Diabetes* March 2013 "Study indicates link between estrogen and body fat storage.

to keep it in check. The excess estrogen signals your body to store more fat cells and grow cancer cells.

Not only does fat store and manufacture estrogen, it also modulates inflammatory responses. Recent evidence indicates that many factors secreted from fat cells are pro-inflammatory.[72]

LCIS

While researching breast cancer types, one type stood out. It is the existence of a pre-cancer called LCIS (Lobular Cancer in Situ). This particular type of cancer is known as a pre-cancer because typically there is no lump felt and no surgery recommended. It is the finding of abnormal cells inside the lobule(s) of the milk duct.

What's interesting is that even though LCIS is found in only 2.5% of breast cancers, they are always estrogen positive and HER2 negative.[73] Additionally, the doctors have no recommendations for prevention with this group, even though there is a 1% risk per year of developing breast cancer. Some doctors may recommend taking tamoxifen or raloxifene if postmenopausal. These drugs reduce the risk to .5% per year. The low amount of risk reduction for cancer may not be worth all the side effects from taking the drug. Monitoring is the only logical thing they can do. A pre-cancerous scenario is a perfect time the S.L.E.E.P. Method can be utilized!

DCIS

Those women who find out they have Ductal Carcinoma in Situ (DCIS) also may be able to utilize the S.L.E.E.P. Method. Ductal carcinoma are abnormal cells isolated inside the milk duct. The cells have not branched out to the rest of the breast or lymph nodes, so they are not

---

[72] http://themedicalbiochemistrypage.org/adipose-tissue.php
[73] Alpers CE, Wellings SR. 1985 *Human Pathology* "The prevalence of carcinoma in situ in normal and cancer-associated breasts."

considered invasive. At this point, the cells are not causing any pain or problems. They appear as little specs or micro calcifications on a mammogram and are not typically felt as a lump.

Approximately 6 to 16% of women are walking around with DCIS and will not die from it, according to autopsies of women who died from other causes. 20 to 24% of these women with detectable DCIS go on to have invasive cancer (infiltrating ductal) up to 25 years after the initial biopsy. Infiltrating ductal cancers typically test positive for estrogen receptors.[74]

If a person does not want that risk, they may decide to get control of these cells now. They do so by choosing surgery, radiation and/or tamoxifen to take it out, shrink it or stop it from growing. This doesn't always stop the invasive breast cancer from coming back in 9% of those who have surgery and radiation, however.

If they are in the low risk category due to a low grade pattern in the milk duct, test estrogen receptor-positive and decide not to have surgery, radiation or take drugs, they may also utilize the S.L.E.E.P. Method for prevention. Even when utilizing medical treatment, certainly, some parts of the S.L.E.E.P. Method can be used simultaneously.

Shrinking Tumors

Prior to breast cancer surgery, surgeons will sometimes give chemotherapy or hormone therapy. The reason they do this, is because the tumor shrinks in 75 to 95% of cases. Shrinking the tumor enables surgeons to have better removal and decrease the likelihood of a full mastectomy. In some cases, they shrink the tumor so much that the surgeon cannot find it. They actually call that surgery a ghostectomy! It seems to me that if they can shrink the tumor and then get a hold of

---

[74] Nielsen M, Jensen J and Andersen 1984 J *Cancer* "Noninvasive cancerous and cancerous beast lesions during lifetime and at autopsy."

the reason it was caused in the first place (estrogen) and put the proper regimen in place, maybe some patients wouldn't need surgery ever!

There are other ways of shrinking tumors. I have heard of a people doing it by having baking soda injected into their tumors (have to go outside the US for this treatment). Another lady used glutathione, a natural antioxidant that prevents damage to cells, to shrink her tumor. Still others have used estrogen detoxification methods and anti-inflammatory methods to shrink their tumors. Some doctors utilize various enzymatic therapies to shrink tumors.

We are so frightened when we find a tumor in our body, we just want to get it out. It makes sense though, that if we can control and shrink the tumor, we may be able make it go away completely and possibly be free from surgery. It is kind of like healing a bad cut in our skin. In this case, we just need to know the right therapy to heal it. Since most breast cancer cases are estrogen receptor-positive, detoxing estrogen would be an appropriate option before, after or in addition to chemotherapy and tamoxifen treatment. Obviously, not all breast cancers are estrogen receptor-positive and may be more difficult to find a proper therapy in time. Also, some breast cancers are invasive and growing fast, so quick action must be taken.

Chapter 6

HORMONES...HOW YOU DOIN?

My Hormone Dilemma

My entire adult life has been plagued by hormonal issues. As a teen, my first indicator that things weren't quite right, was a menstrual cycle fifty-five days long. I kept getting it again and again and it would never go away. I wish I knew then what I know now. This was a sign of lack of progesterone and too much estrogen and or FSH (Follicle Stimulating Hormone).

My mother took me to the doctor who prescribed the birth control pill, which got my cycle in order. Even so, as time progressed, I started having terrible acne and had a hard time keeping weight on. I was so skinny that people called me "string bean" and my brother poked fun at my bird legs. My father thought I was anorexic... literally, so he sent me to a psychiatrist to find out. I did not end up with a diagnosis of anorexia, but the entire experience was just crazy!

In my sophomore year of college, I went off the pill for a while and got unbearable cramps. As I would later discover, those cramps were worse than labor, so back on the pill I went. At around age 30, my sex drive decreased. Right when I was supposed to be at my peak, I was at a low. I had been on the pill for sixteen years. Then at around age 34, I was diagnosed with hypothyroidism, which is related to the endocrine (hormonal) system. At 36, I found a lump in my breast that turned out to be a cyst. At 37, I was diagnosed with Lyme disease and age 43, lumps and cysts found in both my breasts. It was one too many issues for me, so the researcher in me started to chip away at each one of these problems.

I started doing my research in 2002 after I was diagnosed with goiter and hypothyroidism. I was taken aback to learn most of my friends had hypothyroidism, too. Since my endocrinologist wouldn't even so much as recommend a vitamin to help my heart palpitations, I decided to go to various integrative doctors, which is what led me to where I am today.

Little did I know; hypothyroidism is directly linked to breast cancer incidence. Although there are conflicting studies about this link, a study of 102 breast cancer patients in 1996 showed evidence that as much as 46% of breast cancer patients have some kind of thyroid disease. [75] This is why it is so important to get your thyroid tested.

In 2003, my first integrative doctor gave me a prescription for *Armour Thyroid*, which made the heart palpitations go away. *Armour Thyroid* is derived from natural pig hormone. This was some evidence to me that natural hormones can be effective. I stayed on the prescription drug *Synthroid also,* so together, both medications were solving the hormonal imbalance and heart palpitations.

Unfortunately, along my quest to fix my thyroid, I found out more things were wrong with me, which I won't go into here. Because of these issues, I went to a second doctor in 2006. Another hormone saliva panel suggested my progesterone levels were low, so this doctor put me on natural progesterone cream. It seemed to be an almost overnight miracle cure. I was actually able to sleep better, had some increase in sex drive and acne disappeared.

By the time I got to my fourth and current doctor, I was feeling better but still had not cured my thyroid problem- something I am still working on to this day. As I was approaching 40 years of age, my previous doctor had recommended getting a baseline mammogram. I was a little skeptical about mammography so I thought *thermography* would be a

---

[75] Giani C, et al Mar 1996 *J Clin Endocrinol Metab* "Relationship between breast cancer and thyroid disease: relevance of autoimmune thyroid disorders in breast malignancy."

good place to start. I went to Dr. Bruce Rind's office because it was one of two in the area that offered thermography screening.

It turned out that he was the most knowledgeable doctor that I could find regarding women's medical issues. He was a proponent of John R. Lee's, M.D. book, *What Your Doctor May Not Tell You About Breast Cancer*. This book changed my life and gave me insight into what was going on with my hormones. It was also the first book that explained the cause of breast cancer.

Dr. Rind seemed to have more answers than any doctor I worked with. Through thermography screening, he identified my breast lumps. He then introduced me to the steps to get rid of them. That is how I got rid of most my lumps. I followed these steps, which are part of the S.L.E.E.P method.

As you can see, I have been on a path of hormonal imbalance, trying to find good doctors, lots of testing and now recovery. Do any of these problems sound familiar to you? It's good to keep in mind that it took a lifetime to get our bodies to where they are today. It may take a while to get it back on track. Let's start with finding out how your hormones are doing now.

Now that you have heard my story and found out what causes most breast cancer, I am sure you are anxious to take the next step! There are four different testing avenues you can utilize to find out how your hormones are doing. The first two involve reading and are simple screening tests. I would recommend that you take those first. To find out if you have risk areas for breast cancer, you can start by identifying your proestro risk areas in the table. After finding out if you have any or many risk factors, you can take a symptom test to determine if you may have elevated estrogen or not enough progesterone.

After the screening tests, you can take a third type of test- a hormone saliva or urine test from home. You will need to find a doctor who can read these results. The fourth type of screening would be a thermogram. You will need to locate a doctor who can help with a thermography. These four steps will help you identify if you have estrogenic tendencies or any other hormonal imbalances. If you can't do both the urine test and the thermogram, that's okay, I realize it can get a little crazy with the testing sometimes. At least try one to start you in the right direction. I have included more detailed information regarding all of these for you in this section.

If you test high in estrogen and have problem areas identified via thermography, you will want to perform the full S.L.E.E.P. method.

What about the other people who do not test high in estrogen? For breast cancer prevention, these individuals may want to test for inflammation or genetic changes. The HER2 oncogene is a test that is typically done on cancer cells so you can have it done only after you have found out you have cancer. Testing for inflammation can involve allergy testing or blood testing. C-reactive protein is found in the blood. It is generated by the liver and rises and responds when inflammation in the body increases. You can easily have this checked via a blood test. Additionally, you can check for the BRCA gene and other gene mutations anytime. There are several steps in the S.L.E.E.P. method that will benefit those with gene mutations.

Hormonal Relative Risk Factors

Here, I have put together a table where you can easily view hormonal risk factors. I was inspired by a table made by Angela Lanfranchi, M.D., F.A.C.S., Clinical Assistant Professor of Surgery and Joel Brind, Ph.D., Professor of Human Biology and Endocrinology for the Breast Cancer Prevention Institute's Breast Cancer Risks and Prevention 4th edition online booklet[76]. These professors exposed many hormonal risks in their list table. I thought it be helpful to include all the other known hormonal contributors in existence today along with their scientifically proven relative risks.

---

[76] *Breast Cancer: Risks and Prevention* Fourth Edition Angela Lanfranchi, M.D., F.A.C.S and Joel Brind, Ph.D. 2005, 2007

It is about time the amount of risk factors that we have in our lives and their associated level of risk are revealed! You may be surprised, as I was, that all this science exists! Keep in mind that there are ongoing studies, so this table may not be all inclusive or may change over time. But for the first time, you will be able to examine your personal relative risk factors based on most hormonal impacts in your life. Most factors listed increase your risk, but some decrease your risk. Those that decrease your risk will have a negative percentage in the column. Those that increase your risk will have a positive number.

There are several risk factor assessment calculators in existence today. Some are for specific races or populations, which do very little to assess your individual situation. Others are for breast density, which may give a better sense of your current individual current risk. Even so, there is uncertainty in the interpretation of breast density or at what age density matters. Still, other calculators utilize gene traits and hereditary factors to determine risk. Since hereditary is not the main reason why breast cancer is formed and even those with hereditary genes are affected by proestros, it would be more beneficial to utilize a calculator that focuses on the main cause of breast cancer... proestros.

Unfortunately, we cannot create a proestros calculator at this time because of its complexity. Not all risk factors have been tested in combination, so you can't add or subtract them out. For example, for people who drink alcohol, and also have the BRCA gene, risk does not increase very much due to the alcohol. But those who drank and didn't have other risk factors increased their risk significantly.[77]

In the proestros table, if varying effects and risk factors are known, they are accounted for by utilizing high and low percentages within the table. What we are evaluating is the general picture of hormonal risk

---

[77] Willett WC, et al. May 1987 *N Engl J Med* "Moderate alcohol consumption and the risk of breast cancer".

factors in your body over the course of your lifetime. Risk can increase or decrease when risk factors are combined, shortened or lengthened.

We have to be careful to evaluate only the *cause* risk factors. Demographic risk factors are observational and overlap with cause risk factors. In this table I have only included the hormonal influences on risk. For example, age, race and socioeconomic status are observational demographic data risk factors that will have overlap with hormonal influences and cannot be added to the table. Additionally, people with BRCA gene mutations, previous history or family history of breast cancer may have increased or decreased risk in combination with these hormonal risk factors. No matter our age, race or financial status, or previous family history, we are all exposed to proestros.

In this table, relative risk (RR) is the chance of breast cancer incidence associated with one factor compared to women without that particular factor. The percentages in the table are relative risks based on studies or reviews of many studies. Positive RR percentages are associated with breast cancer and negative RR percentages are associated with decreased risk. Here you can highlight the risk factors that apply to you. You may need to refer back to this table as you read further details in Part III to determine what applies to you. The external risk factors listed in the table satisfy the following:

1. Are proven to be estrogenic or anti-estrogenic in human cells
2. Have been found in the human breast
3. Are proven to increase or decrease breast cancer growth in cellular studies

And/or

There are human population studies directly corresponding to an increased or decreased risk to breast cancer.

Even though you cannot add the risk factors up to determine your lowest and highest possible hormonal risk, you can compare risk factors to each other or to the population relative risk. For women, the cumulative lifetime population relative risk (compared to the rest of the population) is approximately 14%. As you go through the table, you can ask yourself how your individual hormonal relative risks compare to the population relative risk. If your risks are higher, you will definitely want to go on to the next screening test.

In some cases, a relative risk factor may not be available, but an odds ratio (OR) is. An odds ratio is similar to a relative risk factor in that it is comparing against two events. An odds ratio calculates the odds of an event happening versus not happening, whereas relative risk calculates the chance of the event happening with exposure relative to no exposure. Relative risk and odds ratios often have similar results. When an odds ratio is used, it will be noted as OR in the table.

BREAST CANCER HORMONAL RISK FACTORS

Risk Factor	Hormonal Effect	Lowest RR	Highest RR	# of Studies	Notes and Studies
External Proestros					
Aluminum	Raises estrogen FSH and LH, increases free iron and invasive properties of BC cells	Iron chelation decreases breast cancer	Unknown	FCS FAS, FHS	78 79 80
Arsenic, inorganic	Increases estrogen	12%	266%	MCS, MAS, FHS	81 82 83
BPA exposure as fetus or infant	Binds to ERs, induces cell growth, accumulates	0%	33% RR in mice	Over 100 CS, MAS, FHS	Banned in baby bottles, 84 85 86 87 88 89

[78] Darbre PD Nov 2013 *J Inorg Biochem* "Effect of aluminum on migratory ad invasive properties of MCF-7 human breast cancer cells in culture".

[79] Darbre PD Nov 2013 *J Inorg Biochem* "Aluminum in breast cancer: Sources of exposure, tissue measurements and mechanisms of toxicological actions on breast biology".

[80] Blaylock RL Mar 2011 www.mercoal.com "New Studies Reveal Alarming Hidden Cause of Breast Cancer".

[81] Garland M et al. Oct 1996 *Am J Epidemiol* "Toenail trace element levels and breast cancer: a prospective study".

[82] Lopez-Carrillo L et al. Oct 2014 *Toxicol Appl Pharmacol* "Arsenic methylation capacity is associated with breast cancer in northern Mexico".

[83] Liu R et al. May 2015 *Epidemiology* "Residential exposure to estrogen disrupting hazardous air pollutants and breast cancer risk: The California Teachers Study".

[84] Soto AM et al. Jun 2013 *J Mammary Gland Biol Neoplasia* "Does cancer start in the womb? Altered mammary gland development predisposition to breast cancer due to in utero exposure to endocrine disruptors".

[85] Lee HR et al. May 2012 *Int J Mol Med* "Treatment with bisphenol A and methoxychlor results in the growth of human breast cancer cells and alteration of the expression of cell cycle related genes, cyclin D1 and p21, via an estrogen receptor-

Risk Factor	Hormonal Effect	Lowest RR	Highest RR	# of Studies	Notes and Studies
Cadmium (urinary)	High amounts increase ER	20%	138%	MCS, MHS	90 91 92 93 94
Copper	High amounts increase ER	Unknown	Anti-copper drug increases BC survival	FHS	95 96 97 98

---

dependent signaling pathway".

[86] Miyawaki J et al. Oct 2007 *J Atheroscler Thromb* "Perinatal and postnatal exposure to bisphenol a increases adipose tissue mass and serum cholesterol level in mice".

[87] Wang L et al. May 2015 *Environ Int* "Accumulation of 19 environmental phenolic and xenobiotic heterocyclic aromatic compounds in human adipose tissue."

[88] Roy D et al. Oct 2015 *Int J Mol Science* "Integrated Bioinformatics, Environmental Epidemiologic and Genomic Approaches to Identify Environmental and Molecular Links between Endometriosis and Breast Cancer".

[89] Yang M et al. Mar 2009 *Arch Toxicol* "Effects of bisphenol A on breast cancer and its risk factors".

[90] Itoh H et al. Jan 2014 *Int J Hyg Environ Health* "Dietary cadmium intake and breast cancer risk in Japanese women: a case-control study".

[91] Strumylaite L et al. May 2014 *Breast Cancer Res Treat* "Association between cadmium and breast cancer risk according to estrogen receptor and human epidermal growth factor receptor 2: epidemiological evidence".

[92] Nagata C, et al. Feb 2013 *Breast Cancer Res Treat* "Cadmium exposure and the risk of breast cancer in Japanese women".

[93] Julin B et al. 2011 *Environ Health* "Relation between dietary cadmium intake and biomarkers of cadmium exposure in premenopausal women accounting for the body iron stores".

[94] Julin B et al. Mar 2012 *Cancer Res* "Dietary cadmium exposure and risk of postmenopausal breast cancer: a population-based prospective cohort study".

[95] Quinin Pan et al. Sep 2002 *Cancer Res* "Copper Deficiency Induced by Tetrathiomolybdate Suppresses Tumor Growth and Angiogenesis."

[96] Jain S et al. Jun 2013 *Ann Oncol* "Tetrathiomolybdate-associated copper depletion decreases circulating endothelial progenitor cells in women with breast cancer at high risk of relapse".

[97] Vahdat Linda et al. Feb 2013 *Weill Cornell Newsroom* "Copper Depletion Therapy Keeps High-Risk Triple-Negative Breast Cancer at Bay."

[98] Martin MB, et al. Jun 2003 *Endocrinology* "Estrogen-like activity of metals in MCF-7 breast cancer cells".

Risk Factor	Hormonal Effect	Lowest RR	Highest RR	# of Studies	Notes and Studies
Diethyl Phthalate (DEP) Monoethyl Phthalate (MEP) Low weight only	Endocrine disruptions via estrogen	120% OR	313% OR for peri-menopausal women	SCS, SAS FHS	99 100 101 102 103
Mercury	Increases ER	Unknown	Unknown	MCS	104 105 106 107 108
Parabens	Estrogenic properties, Enables 4 hallmarks of BC in cells	Unknown	Unknown	SAS, MCS, FHS	109 110 111 112 113

[99] Lopez-Carillo L Apr 2010 *Environ Health Perspect* "Exposure to phthalates and breast cancer risk in northern Mexico".

[100] Sprague BL et al. May 2013 *Breast Cancer Res* "Circulating serum xenoestrogens and mammographic breast density".

[101] Luciani-Torres MG et al. Jan 2015 *Carcinogenesis* "Exposure to the polyester PEET precursor—terephthalic acid induces and perpetuates DNA damage-harboring non-malignant human breast cells".

[102] Oh BS et al. Aug 2006 *Sci Total Environ* "Application of ozone, UV and ozone/UV processes to reduce diethyl phthalate and its estrogenic activity".

[103] Hong EJ et al. Apr 2005 *J Reprod Dev* "Conflict of estrogenic activity by various phthalates between in vitro an in vivo models related to the expression of Calbindin-D9k.

[104] Mohammadi M, et al. 2014 *J Toxicol* "Concentration of cd, pb, hg and se in different parts of human breast cancer tissues".

[105] Byrne C et al. Jan 2013 *J Mammary Gland Biol Neoplasia* "Metals and Breast Cancer".

[106] Egiebor E et al. Oct 2013 *Int J Environ Res Public Health* "The kinetic signature of toxicity of four heavy metals and their mixtures on MCF7 breast cancer cell line".

[107] Martin MB et al. Jun 2003 Endocrinology "Estrogen-like activity of metals in MCF-7 breast cancer cells".

[108] Ionescu JG et al. Dec 2006 *Neuro Endocrinol Lett* "Increased levels of transition metals in breast cancer tissue".

[109] Barr L, Darbre, PD et al. Mar 2012 *J Applied Toxicol* "Measurement of paraben concentrations in human breast tissue at serial locations across the breast from axilla to sternum."

Risk Factor	Hormonal Effect	Lowest RR	Highest RR	# of Studies	Notes and Studies
Perfluor-ooctanoic acid (PCB) and Perfluor-alkylated substances (PFAS)	Enhances effects of estrogen on gene expression	0% OR	659% OR	SAS, 10 HS	Highest in post menopausal women [114] [115] [116]
Pesticide exposure in womb, infancy, puberty or meno-pause	Accumulates in fat tissue, increases estrogen	50%	500%	MCS, MAS, SHS	[33] [34] [35] [36] [37] [38] [39]

[110] Terasaka S et al. May 2006 *Toxicol Lett.* "Expression profiling of estrogen-responsive genes in breast cancer cells treated with alkylphenols, chlorinated phenols, parabens, or bis- and benzoylphenols for evaluation of estrogenic activity."

[111] Darbre PD and Harvey PW Sep 2014 *J Appl Toxicol* "Parabens can enable hallmarks and characteristics of cancer in human breast epithelial cells: a review of the literature with reference to new exposure data and regulatory status."

[112] Wrobel AM and Gregoraszczuk E Nov 2014 *Toxicol Lett* "Actions of methyl-propyl- and butylparaben on estrogen receptor-a and –b and the progesterone receptor in MCF-7 cancer cells and non-cancerous MCF-10A cells."

[113] Braun JN, Just AC et al. Sep 2014 J Expo *Sci Environ Epidemiol* "Personal care product use and urinary phthalate metabolite and paraben concentrations during pregnancy among women from a fertility clinic."

[114] Recio-Vega R et al. Apr 2011 *J Appl Toxicol* "Serum levels of polychlorinated biphenyls in Mexican women and breast cancer risk".

[115] Cohn BA et al. Nov 2012 *Breast Cancer Res Treat* "Exposure to polychlorinated biphenyl (PCB) congeners measured shortly after giving birth and subsequent risk of maternal breast cancer before age 50".

[116] Roy D et al. Oct 2015 *Int J Mol Sci* "Integrated Bioinformatics, Environmental Epidemiologic and Genomic Approaches to Identify Environmental and Molecular Links between Endometriosis and Breast Cancer".

Risk Factor	Hormonal Effect	Lowest RR	Highest RR	# of Studies	Notes and Studies
Polycyclic Aromatic Hydrocarb on (PAH) Benzene, Benzopyre nes	High levels increase ERs and hydrocarbon receptor	48%	240% OR	MCS, SAS, SHS	117 118 119 120 121
Radiation exposure (10 to 450 rads)	DNA cell mutation and increases estradiol and testosterone	36%	1100% Prior to age 20 or during lactation	MHS	35 yr. latency, dose dependen t 122 123 124 125 126 127 128

[117] Guo J et al. May 2015 *Toxicol Letter* "Effects of exposure to benzo[a]pyrene on metastasis of breast cancer are mediated through ROS-ERK-MMP9 axis signaling".

[118] Plísková M et al. Feb 2005 *Toxicol Sci* "Deregulation of cell proliferation by polycyclic aromatic hydrocarbons in human breast carcinoma MCF-7 cells reflects both genotoxic and nongenotoxic events".

[119] Petrallia SA et al. Jun 1999 *Scan J Work Environ Health* "Risk of premenopausal breast cancer in association with occupational exposure to polycyclic aromatic hydrocarbons and benzene".

[120] Gammon MD et al. 2002 *Cancer Epidemiol Biomarkers Prev* "Environmental toxins and breast cancer on Long Island. I. Polycyclic aromatic hydrocarbon DNA adducts".

[121] Modukhovich I et al. May 2015 *Environ Health Perspect* "Vehicular Traffic-Related Polycyclic Aromatic Hydrocarbon Exposure and Breast Cancer Incidence: The Long Island Breast Cancer Study Project (LIBCSP)".

[122] Miller AB et al. Nov 1989 *N Engle J Med* "Mortality from breast cancer after irradiation during fluoroscopic examinations in patients being treated for tuberculosis".

[123] Rhompson DE et al. Feb 1994 *Radiat Res* "Cancer incidence in atomic bomb survivors. Part II Solid tumors, 1958-1987".

[124] Hoffman DA et al. Sept 1989 *J Natl Cancer Inst* "Breast cancer in women with scoliosis exposed to multiple diagnostic x-rays".

[125] Wang JX et al. May 1990 *Int J Cancer* "Cancer Incidence among medical diagnostic X-ray workers in china, 1950 to 1985".

[126] Pukkala E et al. Dec 2012 *Int J Cancer* "Cancer incidence among Nordic airline cabin crew".

[127] Pukkala E et al. Sep 1995 *BMJ.* "Incidence of cancer among Finnish airline cabin attendants, 1967-1992".

Risk Factor	Hormonal Effect	Lowest RR	Highest RR	# of Studies	Notes and Studies
Annual mammo-gram prior to age 50	Increases estradiol and testosterone	1% per mammo gram	43% HR prior to age 30 if BRCA positive	SHS	[129 130 131 132]
Smoking currently or passively	Benzopy-renes arsenic and cadmium increase ERs and may damage cells	19%	608%	MHS	[133 134] worse if smoking prior to 1st FT child or longer duration

Ingested

Alcoholic Beverages	Prevents liver from processing out estrogen, raises free iron	21% three or more drinks per day	150% Two to four drinks per day	MCS, MAS, MHS	Taking Premarin increases risk, BRCA decreases risk, [135 136 137 138]

[128] Grant EJ et al. Nov 2011 *Radiat Res* "Associations of ionizing radiation and breast cancer-related serum hormone and growth factor levels in cancer-free female A-bomb survivors".

[129] Berrington de Gonzalez A, Reeves G 2005 *Brit J Cancer* "Mammographic screening before age 50 years in the UK: Comparison of the radiation risks with the mortality benefits".

[130] Pijpe J et al. Aug 2012 *BMJ* "Exposure to diagnostic radiation and risk of breast cancer among carriers of BRCA1/2 mutations: retrospective cohort study (GENE-RAD-RISK)".

[131] www.mercola.com Dec 2009 "Avoid Routine Mammograms if You Are Under 50"

[132] www.hollitichelp.net/blog/reduce-your-risk-for-breast-cancer/

[133] Catsburg C et al. May 2015 *Int J Cancer* "Active cigarette smoking and risk of breast cancer".

[134] Band PR et al. Oct 2002 *Lancet* "Carcinogenic and endocrine disrupting effects of cigarette smoke and risk of breast cancer".

[135] Willett WC et al. May 1987 *N Engl J Med* "Moderate alcohol consumption and the risk of breast cancer".

Risk Factor	Hormonal Effect	Lowest RR	Highest RR	# of Studies	Notes and Studies
Caffeine	Increases cortisol, may affect estrogen metabolism	-31% for BRCA1 mutation	Increased mortality for BC patients	MCS, MAS, MHS	139 140 141
Sugar intake above 25mg/day	Increases estrogen	87%	187%	MCS, MAS, MHS	142 143
Perfluorinated chemicals (PFOS) i.e. Teflon	Enhance estrogenic effects of estradiol	3%	2830% OR	SCS SHS	144 145 146 147 148 Highest for CYP1A1 and CYP17 gene mutation

136 Key J et al. Aug 2006 *Cancer Causes Control* "Meta-analysis of studies of alcohol and breast cancer with consideration of the methodological issues."
137 Sellers, TA et al. Jul 2001 *Epidemiology* "Dietary folate intake, alcohol and risk of breast cancer in a prospective study of postmenopausal women."
138 *Dr. Susan Love's Breast Cancer Book* p 161 *Stay Young & Sexy*, Susan G Komen, *Breast Cancer Prevention Institute Online Booklet*
139 www.precisionnutrition.com
140 Lowcock EC et al. 2013 *Nutr Cancer* "High Coffee intake, but not caffeine, is associated with reduced estrogen receptor negative and postmenopausal breast cancer risk with no effect modification by CYP1A2genotype".
141 Lehrer S et al. Mar 2013 J *Caffeine Res Coffee* Consumption Associated with Increased Mortality of Women with Breast Cancer".
142 Hu R et al. 2014 *Zhonghua Liu Xing Bing Xue Za Zhi* "Study on the relationship between level of glucose metabolism and risk of cancer incidents".
143 Sulaiman S et al. 2014 *Asian Pac J Cancer Prev* "Dietary carbohydrate, fiber and sugar and risk of breast cancer according to menopausal status in Malaysia".
144 Bonefeld-Jorgensen EC et al. Oct 2011 *Environ Health* "Perfluorinated compounds are related to breast cancer risk in Greenlandic Inuit: a case control study".
145 Ghisari M et al. Mar 2014 *Environ Health* "Polymorphisms in phase I and phase II genes and breast cancer risk and relations to persistent organic pollutant exposure: a case-control study in Inuit women".

Risk Factor	Hormonal Effect	Lowest RR	Highest RR	# of Studies	Notes and Studies
Soy fermented genistein is a main isoflavonoid	blocks estrogen by taking up estrogen receptor site	-77%	-33%	MCS, MAS, MHS	Asian population studies [149] [150] [151]
Soy isoflavonoids extracts, processed or GMO	May increase estrogen signaling at receptor site	Can increase BC, especially when combined with low levels of estradiol	Unknown Post-menopausal exposure may increase risk	MCS, MAS,	[152] [153] [154] [155]

[146] Fenton SE Jun 2006 *Endocrinology* "Endocrine-disrupting compounds and mammary gland development: early exposure and later life consequences."

[147] Bonefeld-Jorensen EC et al. Nov 2014 *Cancer Causes Control* "Breast cancer risk after exposure to perfluorinated compounds in Danish women: a case-control study nested in the Danish National Birth Cohort".

[148] Sonthithai P et al. Aug 2015 J Appl Toxicol "Perfluorinated chemicals, PFOS and PFOA, enhance the estrogenic effects of 17β-estradiol in T47D human breast cancer cells."

[149] Wada K, et al Aug 2013 *Int J Cancer* "Soy isoflavone intake and breast cancer risk in Japan: from the Takayama study".

[150] Woo HD, et al 2014 *Asian Pac J Cancer Prev* "Diet and cancer risk in the Korean population: a meta-analysis".

[151] Mark J Messina and Charles Wood 2008 *Nutritional Journal* "Soy isoflavones, estrogen therapy and breast cancer risk: analysis and commentary".

[152] Hsieh CY et al. Sep 1998 *Cancer Res* "Estrogenic effects of genistein o the growth of estrogen receptor-positive human breast cancer (MCF-7) cells in vitro and in vivo".

[153] Allred CD et al. Sep 2004 *Carcinogenesis* "Soy processing influences growth of estrogen-dependent breast cancer tumors".

[154] Khan SA et al. Feb 2012 *Cancer Prev Res* "Soy Isoflavone supplementation for breast cancer risk reduction: a randomized phase II trial".

[155] Ju YH et al. Jun 2006 *Carcinogenesis* "Genistein stimulates growth of human breast cancer cells in a novel postmenopausal animal model, with low plasma estradiol".

100

Risk Factor	Hormonal Effect	Lowest RR	Highest RR	# of Studies	Notes and Studies
Natural Internal Hormones					
Early menarche age 10 to 12 (mean 13.1)	Increased lifetime estrogen exposure	9%	176%	117 HS	[156][157][175] Each yr. younger, increase premenopausal BC risk by 50 to 67% [158]
Late menarche age 15 to 17	Decreased lifetime estrogen exposure	-12%	-5%	117 HS	[156][157][159] Each yr. older decreases risk
Removal of ovaries with no therapy	Decreased estrogen	-59%	-12%	MHS	[156][157][160]
Early menopause age 35 to 47 (mean 49.3)	Decreased lifetime estrogen exposure	-32%	-12%	117 HS	[156][157][161] Younger decreases risk

[156] http://ww5.komen.org/BreastCancer/RiskFactorsSummaryTable.html
[157] Collaborative Group on Hormonal Factors in Breast Cancer Nov 2012 *Lancet Oncol* "Menarche, menopause, and breast cancer risk: individual participant meta-analysis, including 118 964 women with breast cancer from 117 epidemiological studies".
[158] Iqbal j et al. 2015 *Int J Breast Cancer* "Risk Factors for Premenopausal Breast Cancer in Bangladesh".
[159] Nov 2012 *Lancet Oncol* "Menarche, menopause, and breast cancer risk: individual participant meta-analysis, including 118 964 women with breast cancer from 117 epidemiological studies".
[160] Parker WH et al. May 2009 *Obstet Gynecol* "Ovarian conservation at the time of hysterectomy and long-term health outcomes in the nurses' health study".
[161] Nov 2012 *Lancet Oncol* "Menarche, menopause, and breast cancer risk: individual participant meta-analysis, including 118 964 women with breast cancer from 117 epidemiological studies".

Risk Factor	Hormonal Effect	Lowest RR	Highest RR	# of Studies	Notes and Studies
Late menopause age 53 to 57 (mean 49.3)	Increased lifetime estrogen exposure	5%	30%	117 HS	Each yr. older increases risk by 29%[162] [163]
Exercise 1 to 5 hours per week	Decreases fat cells, lower estrogen cycles, decreases inflammation, increases 2-OHE1/1 ratio16α-OHE	-58%	-6%	Over 50 HS	[164] [165]
No Exercise	Increased estrogen from fat cells	10%	20%	Over 50 HS	[166]
Post-menopausal obesity	Fat tissue becomes source of estrogen, fat causes inflammation	60%	115%	MHS	Higher body mass index, higher the risk [167] [168]

[162] Nov 2012 *Lancet Oncol* "Menarche, menopause, and breast cancer risk: individual participant meta-analysis, including 118 964 women with breast cancer from 117 epidemiological studies".
[163] http://ww5.komen.org/BreastCancer/RiskFactorsSummaryTable.html
[164] Smith AJ et al. May 2013 *Cancer Epidemio Biomarkers Prev* "The effects of aerobic exercise on estrogen metabolism in healthy premenopausal women".
[165] Hildebrand JS et al. Oct 2013 Cancer Epidemiol Biomarkers Prev "Recreational physical activity and leisure-time sitting in relation to post-menopausal breast cancer risk".
[166] http://ww5.komen.org/BreastCancer/RiskFactorsSummaryTable.html
[167] www.cancer.gov and www.mercola.com
[168] Ahn J et al. Oct 2007 *Arch Inter Med* "Adiposity, adult weight change, and postmenopausal breast cancer risk".

Risk Factor	Hormonal Effect	Lowest RR	Highest RR	# of Studies	Notes and Studies
Stressful life events	Cortisol increases or alters estrogen	35% OR	77% OR	MCS, MAS, MHS	Death of a loved one is lowest OR [169] [170] [171] [172] [173]
Maternal Development					
Miscarriage in 1st trimester	Miscarriage is generally due to low estrogen levels	0%	0%	MHS	[174] [175]
Induced Abortion prior to 1st pregnancy (abortion pill or surgical removal)	Increased estrogen without lobule differentia-tion	30%	800%	SAS SHS	[174] [175] [176] [177] The younger (under 18) and more, highest RR

[169] Antonova, Lilia et al. 2011 *Breast Cancer Res* "Stress and breast cancer: from epidemiology to molecular biology".

[170] Simpson ER et al. Sept 1981 *Proc Natl Acad Sci* USA "Estrogen formation in stromal cells of adipose tissue of women: induction by glucocorticosteroids".

[171] Schmidt M, Loffler G 1994 *FEBS Lett* "Induction of aromatase in stromal vascular cells from human breast adipose tissue depends on cortisol growth factors."

[172] Antonova L and Mueller CR Apr 2008 *Genes Chromosomes Cancer* "Hydrocortisone down regulates the tumor suppressor gene BRCA1 in mammary cells: a possible molecular link between stress and breast cancer."

[173] Elzinga B et al Feb 2008 *Psychoneuroendocrinology* "Diminished cortisol responses to psychosocial stress associated with lifetime adverse events: a study among healthy young subjects".

[174] Daling JR et al. Nov 1994 *J Natl Cancer Inst* "Risk of breast cancer among young women: relationship to induced abortion".

[175] Schneider, PA et al. 2014 *The Linacre Quarterly 81* "The breast cancer epidemic: 10 facts".

[176] Bhadoria AS et al. Oct-Dec 2013 *Indian J Cancer* "Reproductive factors and breast cancer: a case-control study in tertiary care hospital of North India".

[177] Brind J et al. Oct 1996 *J Epidemiol Community Health* "Induced abortion as an

Risk Factor	Hormonal Effect	Lowest RR	Highest RR	# of Studies	Notes and Studies
Pregnant to FT in 20s	Increase in estriol	-100%	0	SHS	[175]
Each subsequent pregnancy	Decrease in stage 1 lobules, increase in estriol	-10%	-7%	MHS	[175] Increased risk for BRCA 2 carriers
Delivery or miscarry- age of baby less than 32 weeks	Increased estrogen w/o lobule differentiatio n	22%	111%	MHS	Less than 29 weeks, highest RR [178] [179]
First child after age 35	Increase in % of lobules remaining at stage 1 and exposure to estrogen	10% or 2.3% per yr.	40% or 4.7% per yr.	MHS	26% OR within 5 yrs. after birth [175] [180] [181] [182]
Not breast feeding	Increased estrogen w/o lobule differentiatio n	10%	20%	MHS	[178] [183]

independent risk factor for breast cancer: a comprehensive review and meta-analysis".
[178] Vatten LJ et al. Jul 2002 *Br J Cancer* "Pregnancy related protection against breast cancer depends on length of gestation".
[179] Melbye M et al. May 1999 *Br J Cancer* "Preterm delivery and risk of breast cancer".
[180] Ewertz M et al. Oct 1990 *Int J Cancer* "Age at first birth, parity and risk of breast cancer: a meta-analysis of 8 studies from the Nordic countries".
[181] Susan G Komen website "Breast Cancer Risk Factors Summary Table"
[182] Trichopoulos D et al. June 1983 *Int J Cancer* "Age at any birth and breast cancer risk".
[183] Lambe M et al. Jul 1994 *N Engl J Med* "Transient increase in the risk of breast cancer after giving birth".

Risk Factor	Hormonal Effect	Lowest RR	Highest RR	# of Studies	Notes and Studies
Breast feeding for 13-24 months	Decrease in Stage 1 lobules and estrogen, increase in estriol	-66% OR	-4%	MHS	175 [184] [185]
Breast feeding for 25-48 months	Decrease in Stage 1 lobules and estrogen, increase in estriol	-94% OR	-65% OR	MHS	175 [186] The longer, the lowest
5 or more children	Decrease in Stage 1 lobules and estrogen, increase in estriol	-91%	Add -50% for each child over 5	MHS	176
No Children	No protective Stage 3 or 4 lobules	0	30%	MHS	Long term risk 176 177
Synthetic Hormones					

[184] Collaborative Group on Hormonal Factors in Breast Cancer 2002 *Lancet* "Breast cancer and breastfeeding: Collaborative reanalysis of individual data from 47 epidemiological studies in 30 countries, including 50,302 women with breast cancer from 16 countries".

[185] Xing P, Li J, Jin F Sep 2010 *Med Oncol* "A case-control study of reproductive factors associated with subtypes of breast cancer in Northeast China".

[186] De Silva M et al. Jun 2010 *Cancer Epidemiol* "Prolonged breastfeeding reduces risk of breast cancer in Sri Lankan women: a case control study".

Risk Factor	Hormonal Effect	Lowest RR	Highest RR	# of Studies	Notes and Studies
Birth control during puberty or prior to first FT pregnancy	Progestins increase cell growth	22%	52%	MHS	[187] [188] [189] early onset and highest for BRCA1 carriers
Birth control pill, patch, ring, injection, implant current or recent use for over 8 yrs.	Progestins increase cell growth	20%	104%	Over 55 HS	[187] [190]
Past use (over 4 yrs. ago) of pill, patch ring, injection, implant for any length of time	Progestins increase cell growth	-13%	37%	Over 55 HS	[187] [189]

[187] Collaborative Group on Hormonal Factors in Breast Cancer. 1996 *Lancet* "Breast cancer and hormonal contraceptives: collaborative reanalysis of individual data on 52,297women with breast cancer and 100,239 women without breast cancer from 54 epidemiological studies.

[188] Kotsopoulos J et al. Feb 2014 *Breast Cancer Res* Treat "Timing of oral contraceptive use and the risk of breast cancer in BRCA1 mutation carriers".

[189] Kumle M et al. Nov 2002 *Cancer Epidemiol Biomark Prev* "Use of oral contraceptives and breast cancer risk: The Norwegian-Swedish Women's Lifestyle and Health Cohort Study".

[190] Susan G Komen website "Breast Cancer Risk Factors Table" Birth control pills and breast cancer risk.

Risk Factor	Hormonal Effect	Lowest RR	Highest RR	# of Studies	Notes and Studies
IUD (Progestin) current or recent use	Levonorgestrel has a higher increase in cell growth	22%	200%	MHS	175 [191]
Current or recent (past 3 yrs.) post-menopause hormone replacement	Prempro increases cell growth	25%	140%, 177% if HRT and the pill are used	MHS	1 to 4 yr. latency [192 193 194 195]
DES (Diethylstilbestrol) miscarriage prevention	Synthetic estrogen and endocrine disruptor	27%	35%	10 HS	Taken during 1940-1971 [196]
DES taken by your mother while pregnant	Synthetic estrogen and endocrine disruptor	0%	250%	FHS	Highest over age 40 [197]

[191] Campagnoli C et al. Dec 2005 *J Steroid Biochem Mol Biol* "Pregnancy, progesterone and progestins in relation to breast cancer risk".

[192] Flesch-Janys D et al. Aug 2008 *Int J Cancer* "Risk of different histological types of postmenopausal breast cancer by type and regimen of menopausal hormone therapy".

[193] Ravdin PM et al. Apr 2007 *N Engl J Med* "The decrease in breast-cancer incidence in 2003 in the United States".

[194] Anderson GL et al 2003 *J Am Med Assoc* "Effects of estrogen plus progestin on gynecologic cancers and associated diagnostic procedures: The Women's Health Initiative randomized trial".

[195] Colditz GA Mar 1995 *J Am Med Womens Assoc* "The nurses' health study: a cohort of US women followed since 1976".

[196] Schrager S and Potter B May 2004 *Am Fam Physician* "Diethylstilbestrol Exposure".

[197] http://www.cdc.gov/des/consumers/about/concerns_daughters.html

Risk Factor	Hormonal Effect	Lowest RR	Highest RR	# of Studies	Notes and Studies
Fertility drugs (i.e. Clomid) 12 or more cycles taken or did not become pregnant	Synthetic estrogen	26%	146%	Over 20 HS and ongoing studies up to age 53	[198] [199] 10 to 30 yr. latency

Table Abbreviations:
BC = Breast Cancer
ER= Estrogen Receptors
FT= Full Term
RR= Relative Risk
Yrs. = Years

[198] Brinton LA et al. Apr 2014 *Cancer Epidemiol Biomarkers* Prev "Long-term relationship of ovulation-stimulating drugs to breast cancer risk".
[199] Gennari A et al. Apr 2015 *Breast Cancer Treat* "Breast cancer incidence after hormonal treatments for infertility: systematic review and meta-analysis of population-based studies".

Hormone Balance Test

I used to love taking quizzes in *Cosmopolitan* Magazine, so this brings me back to those days when quizzes were fun. Here's a test you can take by John R. Lee, M.D. As an international authority on hormones and hormone imbalances, Dr. Lee developed this test to help patients find out if their symptoms could be due to a hormonal imbalance. The test has been taken by thousands of women and men worldwide and has proven itself to be remarkably accurate and helpful in identifying different hormone imbalances. If you are a woman, this will help you decide what your next steps may be. Please go to www.JohnLeeMD.com for men test and answers.

Hormone Balance Test – Symptom Checker

Find out if Your Symptoms Are Due to a Hormonal Imbalance
By John R Lee, M.D., Dr. David Zava and Virginia Hopkins

1. Read carefully through the list of symptoms in each group and put a check mark next to each symptom that you have. (If you check off the same symptom in each group that is fine.)

2. Go back and count the check marks in each group. If any group where you have two or more symptoms checked off, there's a good chance that you have the hormone imbalance represented by that group.

3. The more symptoms you check off, the higher the likelihood that you have the hormone imbalance represented by that group. (Some people may have more than one type of hormone imbalance.)

4. It is recommended that you print these pages and use them as reference.

5. Go to the (Women) Answers Section.

HORMONE BALANCE TEST FOR WOMEN

SYMPTOM GROUP 1

□ PMS	□ Insomnia
□ Early miscarriage	□ Painful and/or lumpy breasts
□ Unexplained weight gain	□ Cyclical headaches
□ Anxiety	□ Infertility
TOTAL BOXES CHECKED ☐	

(If you have checked two or more boxes in this group, turn to answers to find out what type of hormonal imbalance you may have.)

SYMPTOM GROUP 2

□ Vaginal dryness	□ Night sweats
□ Painful intercourse	□ Memory problems
□ Bladder infections	□ Lethargic Depression
□ Hot flashes	
TOTAL BOXES CHECKED ☐	

(If you have checked two or more boxes in this group, turn to answers to find out what type of hormonal imbalance you may have.)

110

SYMPTOM GROUP 3

☐ Puffiness and bloating	☐ Cervical dysplasia (abnormal pap smear
☐ Rapid weight gain	☐ Breast tenderness
☐ Mood swings	☐ Heavy bleeding
☐ Anxious depression	☐ Migraine headaches
☐ Insomnia	☐ Foggy thinking
☐ Red flush on face	☐ Gall bladder problems
☐ Weepiness	
TOTAL BOXES CHECKED	

(If you have checked two or more boxes in this group, turn to answers to find out what type of hormonal imbalance you may have.)

SYMPTOM GROUP 4
☐ A combination of the symptoms in #1 and #3

TOTAL BOXES CHECKED

(If you have checked two or more boxes in this group, turn to answers to find out what type of hormonal imbalance you may have.)

SYMPTOM GROUP 5

☐ Acne	☐ Polycystic Ovary Syndrome (PCOS)

☐ Excessive hair on face and arms	☐ Hypoglycemia and/or unstable blood sugar
☐ Thinning hair on head	☐ Infertility
☐ Ovarian cysts	☐ Mid-cycle pain
TOTAL BOXES CHECKED ☐	

(If you have checked two or more boxes in this group, turn to answers to find out what type of hormonal imbalance you may have.)

SYMPTOM GROUP 6

☐ Debilitating fatigue	☐ Unstable blood sugar
☐ Foggy thinking	☐ Low blood pressure
☐ Thin and/or dry skin	☐ Intolerance to exercise
☐ Brown spots on face	
TOTAL BOXES CHECKED ☐	

(If you have checked two or more boxes in this group, turn to answers to find out what type of hormonal imbalance you may have.)

ANSWERS

WOMEN:

1. SYMPTOM GROUP 1
Progesterone deficiency: This is the most common hormone imbalance among women of all ages. You may need to change your diet, get off synthetic hormones (including birth control pills), and you may need to use some progesterone cream. (This is explained in detail in Dr. Lee's books *What Your Doctor May Not Tell You About Menopause and What Your Doctor May Not Tell You About PREMenopause).* And try saliva testing for progesterone and estradiol.

2. SYMPTOM GROUP 2
Estrogen deficiency: This hormone imbalance is most common in menopausal women; especially if you are petite and/or slim. You may need to make some special changes to your diet; take some women's herbs; and some women may even need a little bit of natural estrogen (about one-tenth the dose prescribed by most doctors). (November 1998 pages 1-3) And try saliva testing for estradiol.

3. SYMPTOM GROUP 3
Excess estrogen: In women, this is most often solved by getting off of the conventional synthetic hormones most often prescribed by doctors for menopausal women. You might enjoy this article: Getting off HRT. Once you are on a natural hormone regimen, you may want to get a comprehensive saliva test, Female/Male Saliva Profile III.

4. SYMPTOM GROUP 4
Estrogen Dominance: This is caused when you don't have enough progesterone to balance the effects of estrogen. Thus, you can have low estrogen but if you have even lower progesterone, you can have symptoms of estrogen dominance.

Many women between the ages of 40 and 50 suffer from estrogen dominance. This topic is covered in much detail in Dr. Lee's timeless book *What Your Doctor May Not Tell You About Menopause,* and also in the May 1998 issue of the John R Lee, M.D. Medical Letter. And try saliva testing for Female/Male Saliva Profile 1 or just test for progesterone and estradiol.

5. SYMPTOM GROUP 5
Excess androgens (male hormones): This is most often caused by too much sugar and simple carbohydrates in the diet and is often found in women who also have polycystic ovary syndrome (PCOS). You can find out more about PCOS in *What Your Doctor May Not Tell You About PREMenopause,* as well as the March 1999 issue of the John R Lee, M.D. Medical Newsletter. And try saliva hormone testing for progesterone, estradiol and testosterone.

6. SYMPTOM GROUP 6
Cortisol deficiency: This is caused by tired adrenals, which is usually caused by chronic stress. If you're trying to juggle a job and family, chances are good you have tired adrenals. There are great chapters on restoring your adrenal function in both the Menopause and PREmenopause books, as well as in the July 1998 John R Lee, M.D. Medical Letter. And try saliva hormone testing for the Adrenal function or one of the individual Cortisol tests.

Reprinted by permission from The Official Web Site of Dr. John R. Lee, M.D. (www.JohnLeeMD.com)

So how did you fare? If it is looking a little confusing or daunting, there are other tests you can use to confirm your results. The three types of hormone diagnostics are blood, saliva and urine testing. Checking your hormones through one of these types of tools is imperative as hormone balancing can be tricky and unexpected side effects can happen if you don't use the right hormones or the right levels.

Chapter 7

HORMONE TESTING

Blood Testing

It is important to test your hormones so you know where your problem areas are while balancing. You typically can tell by symptoms if you are on the right track. Blood tests measure systemic circulation of hormone in the blood. When testing the blood, the lab removes and discards the red blood cells, which is where most of the progesterone resides. The part that the lab examines is the plasma or serum, which is the part that is not going to be used by most of the body. Well, that doesn't make any sense, does it? If you are trying to find out progesterone levels, you need the red blood cells.

Not only is the lab measuring unusable progesterone, blood levels can vary depending on the timing of the test. This test only gives a snapshot in time of what is going on at the moment the blood is drawn. Progesterone and other hormones are highly fat soluble and do not stay long in the blood or circulate at steady levels (unless a hormone patch is delivering some hormones to your body).

Another downside to blood testing is that certain hormones cannot be tested. Estriol is not measurable due to its rapid metabolism. The hormone related cancer markers such as 4-methoxyestrone (one of the worst estrogens) do not have blood tests available. For these reasons, blood testing is not a good way to measure hormones, especially progesterone, estriol and 4-methoxyestrone. However, other estrogens can be tested by blood testing.

Saliva Testing

Researchers have been performing saliva testing for years and a number of laboratories offer routine testing. This type of test requires that you put saliva in a test tube at different times of the day, on certain days of the month. Saliva testing offers full panels of sex steroids including progesterone, estrogen, testosterone, DHEA and cortisol, as well as a progesterone to estradiol ratio which can help determine if you have estrogen dominance. The test can be ordered online without a prescription and the cost is quite reasonable. Saliva testing is a good way to find out what your hormone levels are in order to determine if you need any creams to balance out your hormones.

Saliva testing represents the amount of hormone that the tissue actually receives and responds to. Hormones including progesterone, are transported to target tissues from the blood, one of which is the saliva glands. Hence, saliva testing determines how much hormone is entering into the tissues throughout the body.

Saliva testing can be ordered at this website www.johnleemd.com. Here, there are some suggestions from Dr. John R. Lee, M. D's website about which tests to order. However, you may want to finish reading this section before deciding which test to take.

If you are applying a bioidentical hormone cream, saliva testing is a good way to determine whether they are keeping you in balance. Levels in saliva will be higher than normal, especially after the first 3-10 hours of application. After 12-15 hours, the hormone has passed through the body, so it is important to take a saliva test 12-24 hours after applying the cream.

A few years after I was diagnosed with hypothyroidism, my doctors requested that I get my hormones tested. I took three different saliva tests from 2003 to 2007. From these tests I found out I was high in cortisol and low in DHEA and progesterone. My most recent urine test shows the same pattern of high cortisol, (go figure, some things never change) except progesterone is now high.

I did saliva testing of estradiol and progesterone more recently while I was using progesterone cream. The results showed that my estradiol was low. My doctor says I may be nearing menopause, so that could have been why. Regardless, I was experiencing acne and sleepiness so I lowered the progesterone till I felt better. Lowering the progesterone allows the estradiol to rise up a little. Here is a copy of the saliva test I did in December 2012. As you can see, the progesterone appears normal and the estradiol appears low. You will get to see what happens when I do the urine test about two years later.

Hormone Test	In Range	Out Of Range	Units	Range
Estradiol (saliva)		0.6L	pg/ml	1.3-3.3 Premenopausal (Luteal)
Progesterone (saliva)	253		pg/ml	200-3000 Topical, Troche, Vaginal Pg (10-30 mg)
Ratio: Pg/E2 (saliva)	422			Optimal: 100-500 when E2 1.3-3.3 pg/ml

Current Hormone Therapies
25 mg BID topical Progesterone (compounded) (12 hrs Last used). 0.05 mg oral Levothyroxine (T4) (Pharmaceutical) (24 hrs Last used); 15 mg BID oral Armour (glandular thyroid) (Pharmaceutical) (12 hrs Last used);

Interpretation of saliva results can be a little confusing. The normal range for estradiol in women is between 1.5 and 3 picograms per milliliter (pg/ml). The normal range for progesterone is 200 pg/ml or higher. The progesterone and estradiol (pg/E2) ratio is figured by dividing the estradiol into the progesterone. You end up with a number that becomes important in determining if you have estrogen dominance (optimal is between 100 and 500). Certain levels of progesterone are normal for some women, but may be different in others. Reference ranges can change based on stage of life and type of hormone being supplemented. For instance, women in menopause may test lower for estradiol and progesterone. ZRT labs will actually be able to cite what reference range they are using for your individual situation.

Individuals utilizing hormonal creams, will have higher saliva testing results. The progesterone/estradiol ratio can go up to 1000 to 1 in these situations. When you are utilizing a hormone cream, the applied levels of hormone as well as the levels made in the body affect the outcome.

John R. Lee, M.D. and David Zava, Ph.D. recommend saliva testing because it is the only type of test that can accurately measure the biologically active form of the sex hormones.[200] Taking the tests at the appropriate times and days of the menstrual cycle is critical in making sure results are accurate. At this time, saliva testing is not available for hormone metabolites which are excellent risk factor markers for breast cancer.

Urine Testing

Another test you may consider is the urine test. Hormones pass directly through the urine. This test measures hormones your body is dispensing out of the urine and not using, which can be an indicator as to which hormones are high or low. In his book, Dr. Jonathan Wright points to research showing that there may be significant variation in saliva testing, making it less accurate. Urine testing is the method of choice by Dr. Wright and is also recommended by Dr. Lane Lenard, Dr. Bruce Rind and Dr. Joseph Mercola as well as many other integrative doctors. It is not yet routinely used in conventional medicine. More than likely, you will not be able to get your regular physician to order it, due to liability with ordering non-standard tests.

Sex hormones are released in bursts throughout a 24-hour period. They are excreted through the urine. Hormones may not be always consistently concentrated in a single saliva test. Urine may be more accurate because it factors in the bursts and tells us the true 24-hour average. Additional hormones can be tested with the urine test compared to blood and saliva testing. The following hormones can be tested using the urine test: estradiol, estriol, estrone, progesterone,

---

[200] Dollbaum CM and Duwe FJ 7th Annual Meeting of the American Menopause Society, 1997 "Direct Comparison of Plasma and Saliva Levels After Topical Progesterone Application".

118

testosterone, DHEA, 16x-hydroxyestrome, 4-hydroxyestrone, 2-hydroxyestrogen, 2-methoxyestradiol and dihydrotestosterone (DHT). This gives another tool to compute a ratio that can be used in determining breast cancer risk. The 2/16 hydroxyestrone ratio is an important cancer risk factor measurement for hormone related cancers, which can be very important if you want to know where your risks lie.

In his book, Dr. Jonathan Wright recommends having this test done every three to six months while on bioidentical hormone replacement to make sure stable hormone levels have been achieved. The testing is fairly straight forward. Urine testing is done in your home by emptying your bladder into a container for 24 hours. Of course you will have to be at home for this or else you may need to carry a jug around with you, which would not be very practical.

You can either order it yourself online or get it ordered through your doctor. Urine testing ordered through a doctor may be less expensive, which is what I did. My doctor uses Biotek Labs. The cost was around $200. Here is the link to this lab: www.biotek.com. The only thing that I was not completely happy with was Biotek Labs did not test for two of the cancer markers (4MEO1 and 2ME2).

The cost of urine testing without a doctor is a bit higher at around $400. You can go straight to a website and order online yourself without a prescription. I found three companies online who do urinary hormone profiles. They are Meridian Valley Lab, Life Extension and The Wellness Club. Meridian Valley Laboratory does test all breast cancer hormone markers. Here are the websites:

www.meridianvalleylab.com
www.drmyattswellnessclub.com/medicaltests.htm#CompPlus
www.lef.org/Vitamins-Supplements/Blood-Tests/Urinary-Tests.htm

The units used for measurement are different than what is used for saliva testing, so it will be important to find the right doctor who can properly evaluate your test results. Many medical doctors do not realize that blood testing is not a proper tool for full panel hormone testing and do not know how to interpret saliva or urine tests.

Interestingly enough, if you have trouble finding a doctor, there is good news. Dr. Dana Myatt, N.M.D. in Arizona is available to review your results and consult by telephone. Her cost is $60 for 20 minutes. Her website is www.drmyattswellnessclub.com. She is also willing to travel by private plane if necessary and has a Wellness Club Coach for direct visits with patients. Hey that's pretty cool!

My Hormone Test Results

I decided to show you a copy of my urinary hormone tests from 2014 to provide an idea of what results look like. As you can see, I ran a full battery of hormone testing. Some of the same things in my saliva testing show up again, like having high cortisol and low DHEA. I know... you don't have to tell me again that I am stressed out! I am working on that. There is new research in 2012 by Chandrasekhar, K that an herb called ashwagandha, helped people lower cortisol.[201] Ashwagandha is also known to raise DHEA. I tried this herb for more than three months and it seemed to cause breast tenderness. For this reason alone, it is probably not a good idea to take this long term!

We can see from the test that my progesterone is high and my estrogen levels are slightly raised as well. This confirms what I knew about my progesterone levels, but not my estrogen. I thought I might be low in that, which I was not. My doctor says my levels are really good. Everything looks quite even and the progesterone is slightly higher than the estrogen, which is protective. My 16 hydroxyestrone is next to the lowest of the estrogens at 49%, which is an indicator of reduced risk for breast cancer and my 2 hydroxyestrone and estriol is higher (60% and 78% respectively), which is good! Really, I just have a cortisol and DHEA problem, which I will attempt to solve through de-stress methods, anti-cortisol foods and herbs. After this testing, I stopped the estrogen detox protocol and I had already stopped using progesterone cream one year prior to this test!

---

[201] Chandrasekhar K Kapoor, et al Jul 2012 *Indian J Psychol Med* "A prospective, randomized double-blind, placebo-controlled study of safety and efficacy of a high-concentration full-spectrum extract of ashwagandha root in reducing stress and anxiety in adults".

16020 Linden Ave North
Shoreline, WA 98133
www.USBioTek.com
Phone: 206-365-1256
Fax: 206-363-8790

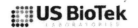

US BioTek
LABORATORIES

Date of Collection: 12-Aug-2014
Reported Date: 28-Aug-2014
Sample Type: Urine

Urine Steroid Hormone Profile   Accession #: 2014063565

All units µg/24hrs

Cortisol/ Cortisol Metabolites

Analyte	Result	Range	0%	20%	40%	60%	80%	100%	%ile	Range Applied
Cortisol	100	30 - 83							89%	Luteal
Tetrahydrocortisol (THF)	1,300	350 - 1,000							92%	Luteal
allo-Tetrahydrocortisol (aTHF)	400	110 - 390							85%	Luteal
Cortisone	180	62 - 160							86%	Luteal
Tetrahydrocortisone (THE)	3,200	1,100 - 3,000							87%	Luteal

17 Hydroxyprogesterone Metabolites

Analyte	Result	Range	0%	20%	40%	60%	80%	100%	%ile	Range Applied
Tetrahydrodeoxycortisol (THS)	59	37 - 110							43%	Luteal
Pregnanetriol (P3)	1,400	450 - 1,500							82%	Luteal

Total 17-hydroxysteroids = aTHF + P3 + THE + THF + THS

Analyte	Result	Range	0%	20%	40%	60%	80%	100%	%ile	Range Applied
Total 17-hydroxysteroids (Total 17HS)	6,300	2,300 - 5,800							86%	Luteal

Test performed by US BioTek Laboratories, 13500 Linden Avenue North, Seattle WA 98133 Ph: 877-318-8728 Fax: 206-363-8790
www.USBioTek.com
CLIA# 50D0965661 Stephen Markus MD Laboratory Director

122

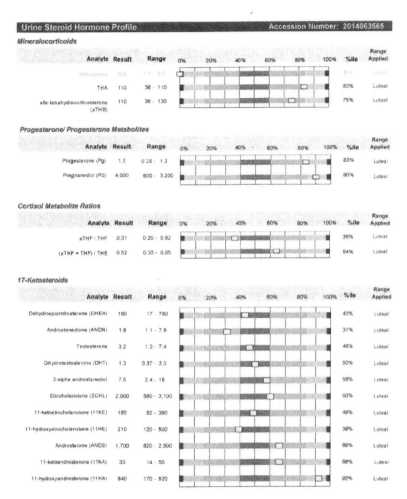

Mineralocorticoids

Analyte	Result	Range	%ile	Range Applied
Aldosterone	N/A	1.3 - 5.5	N/A	Luteal
THA	110	36 - 110	83%	Luteal
allo-tetrahydrocorticosterone (aTHB)	110	36 - 130	75%	Luteal

Progesterone/ Progesterone Metabolites

Analyte	Result	Range	%ile	Range Applied
Progesterone (Pg)	1.2	0.28 - 1.2	83%	Luteal
Pregnanediol (P2)	4,000	600 - 3,200	90%	Luteal

Cortisol Metabolite Ratios

Analyte	Result	Range	%ile	Range Applied
aTHF / THF	0.31	0.20 - 0.82	36%	Luteal
(aTHF + THF) / THE	0.52	0.33 - 0.65	84%	Luteal

17-Ketosteroids

Analyte	Result	Range	%ile	Range Applied
Dehydroepiandrosterone (DHEA)	160	17 - 780	43%	Luteal
Androstenedione (ANDN)	1.8	1.1 - 7.8	31%	Luteal
Testosterone	3.2	1.3 - 7.4	46%	Luteal
Dihydrotestosterone (DHT)	1.3	0.37 - 3.3	50%	Luteal
3-alpha androstanediol	7.5	2.4 - 16	58%	Luteal
Etiocholanolone (ECHL)	2,000	880 - 3,100	60%	Luteal
11-ketoetiocholanolone (11KE)	180	82 - 390	49%	Luteal
11-hydroxyetiocholanolone (11HE)	210	120 - 500	39%	Luteal
Androsterone (ANDS)	1,700	620 - 2,500	86%	Luteal
11-ketoandrosterone (11KA)	33	14 - 50	66%	Luteal
11-hydroxyandrosterone (11HA)	640	170 - 520	92%	Luteal

123

Urine Steroid Hormone Profile   Accession Number: 2014063565

Total 17-Ketosteroids = DHEA + ECHL + ANDS + 11HA + 11HE + 11KA + 11KE

Analyte	Result	Range	0%	20%	40%	60%	80%	100%	%ile	Range Applied
Total 17-ketosteroids (Total 17KS)	4.800	2.200 - 7.400							61%	Luteal

Anabolic Catabolic Ratio

Analyte	Result	Range	0%	20%	40%	60%	80%	100%	%ile	Range Applied
Anabolic 17KS / Catabolic 17HS	0.76	0.72 - 1.7							18%	Luteal

Androgen Ratios

Analyte	Result	Range	0%	20%	40%	60%	80%	100%	%ile	Range Applied
DHT / Testosterone	0.41	0.23 - 0.67							49%	Luteal
Androsterone / Etiocholanolone	0.85	0.46 - 1.1							67%	Luteal

Estrogens/ Estrogen Ratios

Analyte	Result	Range	0%	20%	40%	60%	80%	100%	%ile	Range Applied
Estrone (E1)	13	3.7 - 20							70%	Luteal
Estradiol (E2)	5.4	1.2 - 6.6							77%	Luteal
Estriol (E3)	13	2.7 - 15							78%	Luteal
EQ = E3 / (E1 + E2)	0.59	0.26 - 1.0							64%	Luteal
2-hydroxyestrone (2OHE1)	8.6	2.9 - 16							60%	Luteal
4-hydroxyestrone (4OHE1)	0.70	0.27 - 1.3							51%	Luteal
16-hydroxyestrone	4.4	1.8 - 9.8							49%	Luteal
2-methoxyestrone (2MeOE1)	3.0	1.1 - 6.6							54%	Luteal
4-methoxyestrone (4MeOE1)	<0.45	0.40 - 2.5							<18%	Luteal
Sum of Estrogens	46	21 - 72							67%	Luteal
2MeOE1 / 2OHE1	0.35	0.22 - 0.70							47%	Luteal

Page 3

Chapter 8

HEREDITARY AND GENE TESTING

You won't be able to find out if you have ER+ or HER2+ markers unless you have a breast tumor to test. You can, however, find out if you have one of the hereditary genes in advance.

Tests are available to determine if genetic defects play a part in your cancer risk. Testing positive for BRCA1 or BRCA2 gene mutations does *not* necessarily mean you will get breast cancer, but it does increase your risk. BRCA1 and BRCA2 mutations account for five times the normal risk of breast cancer and 10 to 30 times the risk of ovarian cancer. BRCA mutations account for 45% of breast cancers that are deemed hereditary, and about 1.5 to 5% of all breast cancer. BRCA genes are tumor suppressor genes found in all humans.

Typically, people without breast cancer don't test for this gene unless they know they have a relative with breast, ovarian, fallopian tube or primary peritoneal cancer. The reason why is because there are over 700 mutations possible in BRCA genes, which makes it more expensive to find. The other reason why this testing is not typically recommended is because only .23% or less of people without breast cancer test positive for this gene.[202]

Myriad Genetics patented the methods to diagnose BRCA mutations. Controversy over high testing prices and an inability to get research confirmation from other labs led to a lawsuit. As of December 2012, isolated genes remain patentable in the US. Some of the arguments against patents on genes say that they stifle innovation by preventing others from conducting cancer research and limit options for cancer patients seeking genetic testing. Additionally, the case against patents

---

[202] The American Society of Breast Surgeons www.breastsurgeons.org

argues that patents are not valid because companies cannot patent genetic information that is intrinsic to all humans. It is worth noting that Myriad Genetics is a $500-million-dollar company. It doesn't take much to imagine the conflict between money and health in the breast cancer industry.

Hereditary testing is a blood drawn test that can cost between $300 and $3500, depending on how in-depth the workup is. There is a limited test that looks for three mutations common for Ashkenazi Jews (loosely defined as Jews of central and eastern European lineage), as well as a mutation shared in common with another relative with breast cancer. The full test will search out the known 700 mutations in this gene. Many insurance plans cover this test, but there are a few disheartening cases where insurance providers raised rates or denied claims due to the results of the test. To that end, the federal Genetic Information Nondiscrimination Act of 2008 protects those undergoing genetic testing.

You can seek testing through a genetic counselor, your primary care doctor or your gynecologist. Genetic counselors for cancer are available throughout the US. You can go to http://www.cancer.gov/cancertopics/genetics/directory for a searchable directory of counselors.

Okay, so you decide to do this test and you test positive. Now what? Preventative action recommended for this scenario is to close monitoring, chemoprevention or even removal of your breasts. Close monitoring usually involves regular mammograms. This is conflicting because BRCA positive women's breast tissue is typically denser, making it harder for mammography to detect tumors. In addition, mammograms detect less than half the breast cancers in BRCA mutation carriers.[203] Other options for monitoring include ultrasound and MRI, which have limitations on their own. Ultrasound waves

---

[203] Kriege M et al. 2004 *N Engl J Med* "Efficacy of MRI and mammography for breast cancer screening in women with a familial or genetic predisposition".

weaken as they pass through tissue. The more tissue present, the more difficult it will be to read deep within the breast. MRIs cannot always distinguish between cancerous and non-cancerous areas in the breast and they do not detect micro-calcifications, which can indicate breast cancer.

There is another tool not as well-known, called thermography. It can also be used for monitoring. It has limitations for deep tissue, but it does not include any increased risk of cancer growth as there is when using x-rays. Be aware that there will be a need to monitor the pelvic area as well for other cancers associated with the BRCA mutation and thermography can do that as well.

As mentioned previously, BRCA1 positive, estrogen-receptor negative tumors also respond to estrogen reducing treatments. If you test positive for this mutation, why not try some proestros reduction steps now? This not only reduces risk for breast cancer, it prevents other estrogen sensitive cancers, including cancers BRCA mutations are known for.

It may seem excessive to have your breasts removed, but to many it may be a life saver. If Angelina Jolie can do it, why can't you? It may be that removal will be less traumatic than having to undergo lumpectomy, radiation and chemo. In fact, mastectomy gives you a 90% risk reduction of subsequent breast cancer. Then you will still have your ovaries to contend with.

Personally, now that I know how to control proestros going into my body, I would do these scientifically proven methods instead and diligently utilize thermography and ultrasound. Some of us may not want to deal with all that discipline and worry, which makes this a very personal decision.

Chapter 9

BREAST CANCER DETECTION

One day, it happened to me. I experienced the breast cancer scare. My husband found an enlarged lump on my right breast-thank goodness for husbands feeling us up! I quickly called the OB-GYN and went straight to the doctor's office. They wrote up a slip for me to go to the radiology unit. I was amazed to see so many women wearing pink hospital gowns waiting for a mammogram, just like me. It made it clear to me how big a health condition breast cancer is.

I should have been checking myself, but no...I hadn't been. If I had known that 80% percent of breast cancer is detected by regular self-exam, maybe I would have been more diligent. A monthly breast self-exam should have three steps: a visual exam in front of a mirror, exam while in the shower and exam while lying down. If you are not in menopause, it should be done about one week after the start of your period.

Aside from self (and husband assisted!) exams, what are the other possible ways to detect breast cancer? Clinical exams are typically performed at the OB-GYN, so you only get checked once a year this way. Numerous health organizations, including the US Preventive Services Task Force and American Cancer Society recommend that this be performed annually at your physical exam. However, research has not found that clinical exams reduce breast cancer deaths.

Mammography is the chief method used for screening since the late 1970s. We are informed that mammography decreases the mortality rate and encouraged to undergo yearly mammograms. However, there is mounting evidence that this procedure may not be all it is alleged to be. In fact, The Canadian Chief Medical officer, Otis Brawley, admitted that "American medicine has overpromised when it comes to screening. The advantages to screening have been exaggerated." Some doctors believe that radiation exposure can actually speed up cell production for problem area cells. There is actually a 1% increase risk for breast cancer for each year you receive a mammogram if you start at age 40.[204] [133] For those with BRCA gene mutation, the risk goes up if mammograms are performed annually starting before age 30.[205]

Even with this new thinking about mammography, doctors are recommending testing annually. There are still studies that show it may be worthwhile for a few people. A 2010 study showed that 2.1 deaths were prevented out of 200,000 people. Eight trials of mammography saw a more impressive number for women aged 50 to 69. Each one demonstrated that there was one fifth fewer breast cancer deaths with those women that were screened.

Knowing the low prevention rate for women under 50, I wasn't convinced to get a mammogram the first time we found a lump. I declined a mammogram and went first with an ultrasound on my right breast. The radiologist took a look at it and knew right away that it was a cyst. There! No mammogram needed to tell me what that lump was!

The nurses were not very happy with me for turning down the mammogram. I wondered to myself if they were paid for each mammogram performed. It felt like peer pressure. "Come on, everybody's doing it". "There is not much radiation". When it comes to personal decisions about a women's body, peer pressure is invasive and totally inappropriate. Why would anyone want to have so much influence on my body? You can argue that they just want to help, but after all that stress, the mammogram wasn't needed and there was nothing I could do about a cyst...or so they believed.

[204] Berrington de Gonzalez A, Reeves G 2005 *Brit J Cancer* "Mammographic screening before age 50 years in the UK: Comparison of the radiation risks with the mortality benefits".
[205] Pijpe J et al. Aug 2012 *BMJ* "Exposure to diagnostic radiation and risk of breast cancer among carriers of BRCA1/2 mutations: retrospective cohort study (GENE-RAD-RISK)".

In 2009, the US Preventative Services Task Force (USPSTF) lowered the recommendation for annual screenings for patients before age 50. The USPSTF is an independent group of national experts in the prevention of disease with a focus on evidence-based medicine. Most of its sixteen members are practicing clinicians who volunteer their time and effort. The weird thing is, I never heard of them or their recommendation that I don't need to do annual testing prior to age 50. Have you? For some reason the American Cancer Society still recommends annual mammograms from age 45 to 55 and every other year after age 55.

Here I was in my 30s with a lump and being told that it is a personal decision. When I made that decision, I was made to feel bad about it. The USPSTF recommends mammography testing every two years for women age 50 to 74. So being that I am younger than 50, I can wait till I am 50 to do it every other year. New York and Virginia recently passed laws requiring women with dense breasts to be informed they may need to seek alternative screening methods which include ultrasound, MRI and thermography. These recommendations indicate that we are moving away from mammography as the sole tool for detection.

The second time I found an unusual lump was at my fourth integrative doctor's office. There, I was encouraged to get a mammography. I figured since I was a little over 40 years old, I probably should do something, but wasn't comfortable with mammography because of the associated radiation exposure and potential to actually cause cancer, prior to age 50. After researching options, I found out about thermography and decided to try it under the guidance of Dr. Bruce Rind.

Thermography

Thermography is digital imagery of temperatures on the breast surface using infrared thermal imaging (DITI), to produce colored or black and white images. The patterns reflect metabolic activity inside the breasts and neighboring lymph nodes. Much like an infrared camera can detect heat loss within your home, the thermogram can detect differences in temperatures down to a tenth of a degree Celsius and identify problem areas. Benign conditions such as cysts and lumps tend to show no thermal activity. Thermography helps differentiate problem areas from non-problem areas and gives us a tool for assessment. Certain thermal patterns have become associated with breast problems. For instance, if there is inflammation of any sort, regardless of the cause, the inflammation creates heat and is detected by the thermography equipment. Even more important than assessment, thermography gives us a tool for feedback after a problem has been found and the patient has worked to resolve it.

Thermography was given a bad name after it was being used in the 1960s. Anyone with a thermal imager was allowed to perform *Medical Digital Infrared Imaging*, leading to outrageous claims and "findings" that were easily challenged and discredited by medical professionals. There were no standards for equipment and no requirements for the qualification and certification of medical thermologists. Interpretation was incredibly subjective as no acceptable protocol was established for the imaging user.

These were the perfect ingredients for the discrediting and failure of thermography within the medical field. In addition, the fear of having a new technology take profit from certain equipment makers, medical associations and doctors is a great deterrent to progress. Today, there are advancements in infrared technology as well as defined standards and practices have been established.

One important change to breast thermography when using a FLIR® type camera is the *cold challenge*. The first thermogram is taken at a normal temperature and the second is taken after cooling down the body significantly. This makes cancer cells stand out, as they do not cool down as quickly as regular cells, partially because cancer cells have increased blood flow around them. In addition to this technique, a camera specifically made for the human body, the Meditherm® System, can detect even smaller temperature changes than the FLIR camera and can be used anywhere on the body.

When timed correctly, the thermogram can detect irregular cells on the breast surface. This does not necessarily mean these cells are cancerous, but they could later become cancerous. **It is critical to understand that thermography is not a cancer confirmation tool such as a biopsy.** It is a problem area detection tool.

One practice that aids thermography screening is timing the procedure properly within your cycle. Estrogen tends to be lower right after your period. If you get thermograms done routinely, you want to make sure you are getting them done within five days of the end date of your cycle, when estrogen is lowest. If you go prior to your period, everything may be swollen or exaggerated and higher temperature, due to higher estrogen levels.

I stood there watching as the thermography monitor in front of me was showing all kinds of dark green, yellow and red colors against a pale blue background of the rest of my body. You didn't have to have a trained eye to see it didn't look good. There was a dark green area on the lower left breast and large areas of darkness on the chest on that same side. The thermogram found a huge lump in my lower left breast, which I could then feel. That was pretty scary! Nothing like a little fear to get you doing stuff you never thought you would do. If only all women got thermograms- it might motivate them to be more proactive.

The doctor quantifies the exam based on healthy results. On a scale of 1 to 5, 5 being the worst, I got a 4.5 on the left breast and a 4 on the right. Without hesitation, my doctor recommended a breast treatment protocol for prevention and a mammogram to determine if I may have had cancer.

After seeing these results, I was convinced to go get a mammogram. I figured if anything, it would be good to have a baseline mammogram on file. I had the mammogram done right after my first thermogram. Luckily for me, the results came back negative. I couldn't believe that the mammogram did not see that huge lump that I could feel and see in the thermogram, but I can only assume the lump was not cancerous since it didn't detect it.

In essence, I learned that mammograms catch cancer once it has already developed. By the time it is found, it may be too late. Many women go into panic mode and may not have much time for reduction strategies before going into surgery and chemo and radiation treatment. If only people knew more about thermography testing.

Another tool that is being used in detection is 3D mammogram technology. According to the Vice President of the National Breast Cancer Coalition, 3D mammogram technology is new and should not be used outside of a clinical trial. When I looked into the research, it appears that it is still undergoing clinical trials as of this publication. The research is being funded by Hologic, the manufacturer of the 3D machine, which may present a conflict of interest.

After my experiences with all detection tools available, I am in favor of regular thermograms. You really can't go wrong- there are no health risks to the procedure and if something comes up, you can still get your mammogram or ultrasound.

In addition to my doctor's office (uses FLIR camera), Center for Health and Healing, I have located a company that performs thermography (using Meditherm camera system) in multiple locations across the US. There are currently 29 locations in Virginia, 18 in Maryland and Washington DC, 24 in Wisconsin, 26 in Chicago and one in the Florida Keys.

The Longevity Center
888-580-0040
www.longevitythermography.com

The Center for Health and Healing
800 S. Frederick Ave Suite 202
Gaithersburg, MD 20877
301-971-4325

My Thermograms

I was a little apprehensive at first, but I made the decision to share my thermogram photographs. What is the point of this whole book, if you can't see the results you can achieve? Next you'll see four black and white thermograms over the course of two and a half years of doing the S.L.E.E.P. Method. If you look at each photo, you can see that the dark areas get subsequently lighter. The lower left lump area could no longer be felt by hand and had faded significantly in the 2013 pic. The reason why the veining starts out dark is because tissue tends to be warmer where there is estrogenic activity.

134

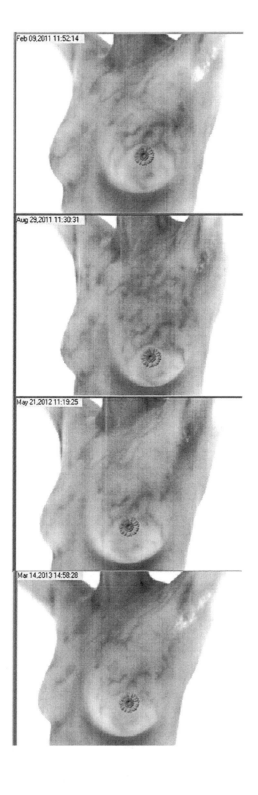

The color images below show my first thermogram on the left (February 2011) and then my second on the right (October 2011). (If you are reading a black and white version of this book, you will not be able to see these visible results.) Eight months had passed and there is not much difference between the two. The green area (dark area at circle 2) on the lower left breast is the lump that has increased in size. The patch on my chest (circle 4) has also increased in size. The overall temperature has also increased. The green patches on the right breast did decrease slightly.

Why hadn't much changed? I was practicing most of the S.L.E.E.P. Method, but I did not have my IUD removed as of yet. This demonstrates my first-hand experience of how strong IUD progestin hormones are and how little estrogen detoxification does against them while they are going into our body simultaneously. Still, there was some improvement in the black and white photos as seen above, so that gave me some hope.

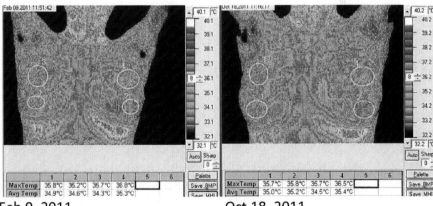

Feb 9, 2011   Oct 18, 2011

After having the IUD removed in January 2012, progress was made in both breasts on the thermogram (below right) in May 2012, seven months later. Blue is starting to be my favorite color! The lower left and right green areas have virtually disappeared; overall green pattern is reduced and nipple temperature difference is reduced. Physically, I could no longer feel the lump on the lower left. My rating was downgraded to a 3.5. What a relief ...sort of- I still had work to do on the upper left breast area. I believe this green area is the lymph that is congested and may take longer to excrete estrogens. I should have never been given an IUD knowing that I had high risk factors, namely starting synthetic birth control as a teenager, using birth control for more than eight years and with no protective risk factors such as having children at a young age.

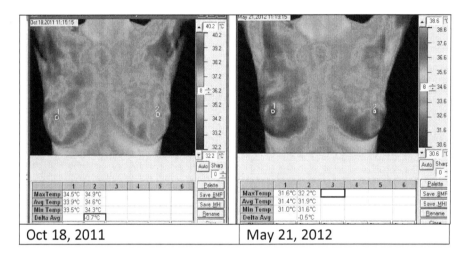

Oct 18, 2011	May 21, 2012

It's important to note that my results are not unique. I've seen other women who have done this too, with even better thermography results than I had. It is simply amazing that we can actually chart our progress with thermography! This is proof that IUD removal was the right thing for me to do- I was already at high risk. The S.L.E.E.P. Method helped me get rid of a lump and lower inflammation in many areas of my chest. It has also helped other women who were not using patentable hormones have similar results, and it can for you too!

Chapter 10

FINDING A DOCTOR

Finding a doctor was the most frustrating part of healing. As you can see, I went through four of them. Having a regular general practitioner has been imperative for routine exams, illness, and emergencies, so of course I started with a visit to a medical doctor to establish myself as a patient. I made sure he was close to home.

The next thing I did was find an integrative doctor who supported my path to healing through both natural and medical methods. Even my general practitioner seemed interested in some of the supplements I was utilizing. Many medical doctors are starting to be open to alternative solutions, says the 2012 Mayo Clinic Breast Cancer Book.

"In a government funded survey, almost 40 percent of adults interviewed reported using some form of complementary or alternative medicine, including natural and herbal products and therapies deep breathing, meditation, chiropractic care, yoga and massage, among others. Doctors and scientists also are taking a keener interest in studying the safety and potential benefits of nontraditional therapies and a number of rigorous research studies are underway."

So, you can ask your general practitioner if he/she performs the following:

1 Vitamin D3 blood testing
2 Hormone urine testing and result evaluation
3 Iodine urine testing
4 Breast thermography
5 Formulate a prescription hormone cream by working with a compounding pharmacy

Your doctor may not have had much experience with bioidentical hormones but may be willing to try it. If that is the case, you can put him/her in touch with your local compounding pharmacy. Sometimes pharmacies hold seminars for doctors and patients willing to learn the latest on hormone replacement.

Seminars can be found at:

www.tahomaclinic.com
www.bioidenticalhormonesociety.com

The terminology for clinicians outside so-called "mainstream" medicine has evolved over the last few decades. What started out as "natural" medicine in the 1990s, has branched out to complementary, alternative, and integrative medicine. I have included definitions to help decipher today's terminology and help you figure out what style you may like.

Complementary usually refers to treatments used in conjunction with conventional medicine. These techniques help if you are already receiving treatment for breast cancer, but can also help to reduce stress for prevention of breast cancer. These type of treatments include meditation, massage, yoga, progressive relaxation, hypnosis and music therapy. Supplements may also be considered complementary and can be used in conjunction with conventional medicine. These supplements may include vitamins, herbs and certain foods.

Osteopaths are primary care physicians that offer a type of complementary medicine. *Osteo* comes from the Greek word for bone. Typically, these practitioners are chiropractors, specializing in internal medicine, surgery, pediatrics or pathology. They are different from regular medical doctors in that they concentrate on the whole person and favor a preventative approach. Many can prescribe drugs and hormone creams.

Alternative refers to treatments used in place of traditional medicine. However, many people use the term *alternative medicine* when referring to either complementary or alternative. Alternative medicine is any practice that has healing effects of medicine but is not based on evidence gathered with the scientific method. Alternative medicine believes in energies and folk medicine. They may use herbs for healing, Chinese medicine, acupuncture, Reiki, homeopathy and naturopathy.

Naturopathy is based on the belief that when the body is given the correct natural materials and energies, it has the power to heal itself. Naturopathic practitioners are split into two groups, traditional naturopaths and naturopathic physicians. Traditional naturopaths tend to focus on one treatment modality such as acupuncture or nutrition or botanical remedies.

Naturopathic physicians (NDs) use the principles of naturopathy within the context of conventional medical practices. NDs receive a four-year graduate level school with less emphasis on drugs and surgery and more on nutrition, bioidentical hormones, botanical remedies, homeopathy, acupuncture or other non-toxic therapies. The main idea is to treat the root cause of the illness, not just the symptoms. NDs emphasize prevention, lifestyle changes and wellness and will take more time to understand your individual situation.

Integrative medicine is the fairly new concept where complementary and conventional medical interventions are used together to treat the whole person, not just the disease. These doctors must have a medical degree but may also have a secondary education in complementary or naturopathy methodologies. Some complementary therapies might be more preventative: using supplements, vitamins or mind/body techniques. Some of these therapies are being studied at the Mayo Clinic. All my doctors have been integrative doctors.

There are several places you can turn to find an integrative or alternative doctor. Here are a few web sites:

1 The American Association of Naturopathic Physicians at
www.naturopathic.org 866-538-2267

2 American College for Advancement of Medicine (ACAM) – This is the largest and oldest.
www.acamnet.org 888-439-6891

3 International College of Integrative Medicine (ICIM)
www.icimed.com   866-464-5226

4 American Academy of Environmental Medicine (AAEM)
www.aaemonline.org 316-684-5500

5 American Osteopathic Association
www.osteopathic.org 800-621-1773

6 Bioidentical Hormone Initiative
www.bioidenticalhormoneinitiative.org/content/locate-bhrt-doctor

7 Academy of Integrative Health and Medicine
www.aihm.org (218) 525-5651

If you are pretty sure you are going to need a hormone cream, you can contact a local compounding pharmacy who can then refer you to a doctor who knows how to read hormone tests and prescribe a cream for you. References for compounding pharmacies are located in Step P section of this book.

PART III

TAKING ACTION

Chapter 11

THE S.L.E.E.P. METHOD

Now that we've established the range of causes and diagnostic tools available, it's time to take real steps to prevent and reduce the impact breast cancer has in your life. If we could only read the future to see what we are facing in terms of breast cancer, then perhaps we would be inspired to do something to stop it. Thermography testing is what gave me inspiration and hopefully, will for you too.

Some people have the perseverance to make an entire life change. Some are willing to change a few things. Either way, making any change at all helps not only you, but the people that surround you. Whether we realize it or not, we are a role model and our example encourages others. Our health is in our hands. We are the final decision maker. We are the ones who care more about our body than anyone else. We have the control over it and we are what we eat and what we put on it.

To make the concept of change easier and to speed up the road to put breast cancer to sleep, I have narrowed it down to five easy steps, which I call the S.L.E.E.P. Method. The S.L.E.E.P. Method is a compilation of the best research. Integrative doctors including Dr. Bruce Rind, Dr. Joseph Mercola, Dr. Jonathan Wright, Dr. Lane Lenard and Dr. John R. Lee, M.D who have proven in their own practices that various methods in these steps work. Dr. Susan Love and the Mayo Clinic, as well as most medical doctors also recommend some of the methodologies in these steps. These are the steps I took and many other patients have taken to get rid of or prevent breast lumps.

Each letter in the S.L.E.E.P. Method stands for one step to keep breast cancer asleep. Supplements, lifestyle, eating well, eliminating proestros and progesterone supplementation are the pillars of this approach.

Each step drives at a singular purpose: to eliminate the one thing that causes the vast majority of breast cancer cases- **proestros**.

After having my IUD removed and following this protocol, my larger lumps disappeared after three months (seven months between thermograms)! I firmly believe that lumps can be reduced within a four-month time period, once all steps are being followed. If doctors can reduce or get rid of tumors in three to four months using drugs, certainly we can reduce lumps that have not (yet) become cancerous!

My doctor, Dr. Rind, has been able to help many women diagnosed with breast cancer reduce their tumors. One women came in after one month of doing this method and found out her lump was significantly reduced. Another woman reduced all her lumps by high dose vitamin D alone!

Our body treats many foreign objects like an estrogen. These foreign objects (proestros) promote estrogens that build up over time in our bodies and wreak havoc. It may not be now...but it may be sooner than you think.

These proestros cause breast cancer, among other types of cancer. So the number one goal when trying to prevent or get rid of cancer is to slow the body's burden of proestros, decrease estrogen intake and detoxify it out of the body. The S.L.E.E.P. protocol is designed to do just that.

Since approximately 25% of breast cancer is caused by the HER2 and hereditary gene mutations, I will be addressing prevention tips in parts of this protocol that may also help in those situations. Some of the supplements and foods are scientifically shown to help those with other types of pre-dispositions to breast cancer, since they directly attack cancer in general. We will start with supplements.

Chapter 12

S IS FOR SUPPLEMENT

Rediscovering Natural Remedies

When I first started researching breast cancer, I was surprised to discover how much controversy exists surrounding research, detection and treatment. There is an incredible amount of push and pull between the medical and naturopathic communities. Our medical environment today has changed quite a bit from many years ago. Natural remedies were the norm because that's what was available. Synthetic medicine has taken the lead since the discovery of cures such as antibiotics. Due to the demand for cures, research is being performed on both synthetic medicines and natural remedies. I was able to easily find the science involved that complements the road to breast cancer prevention.

Unfortunately, natural remedies frequently are not given much credence because many times studies are not funded well, or their length or number of case studies may be limited. As research in this area becomes more robust and exhaustive, natural medicine is coming back into the conversation. Those people with medical issues that have no medical cure, still may not be offered alternative solutions at the doctor's office, but they may be able to find other solutions, other places.

More and more we are hearing about the dangers or negligence in taking herbs and supplements. Sorting through natural cures can be a mess. Typically herbs or supplements are not approved by the FDA, so we have no way of knowing if the amount of testing and quality of the product is sufficient. We are left having to do the research on our own.

How I came to start looking at natural remedies is a bit unusual. Many years ago, my cat had diabetes and irritable bowel syndrome (IBS) and the IBS was not responding to any regular treatments. I was cleaning up messes all over the house and giving insulin shots. (Now, I ask myself why a pet owner would go through this.) I was at a loss as to what to do. I figured, ok, it's a cat, I'm tired of cleaning up the messes, so I'll devise some alternative solutions. I decided to try ground alfalfa and probiotics mixed into his food because they are known to help digestive issues and voila! My cat's irritable bowel disappeared. This proved to me that natural remedies can actually have an impact. From then on, I began seeing alternative and natural medicine in a different, more credible light.

This led me to try advice from an alternative veterinarian. She showed me where I could get recipes to make homemade raw cat food, which included vitamins, rice and raw ground turkey. I fed this homemade concoction to my cat every day. Eight months later, I was startled in the middle of the night by the sound of a cat making insistent, unusual howling noises. Needless to say, I rushed him to the emergency pet hospital where they discovered he didn't need insulin shots anymore. His diabetes was cured! Did you know cat diabetes could be cured? I didn't!

Well thank goodness for the insulin shots that kept him going until he was cured. And thank goodness for healthy eating, probiotics and ground alfalfa. I saw first-hand how in its basic form; the body has the ability to cure itself if it is given the right ingredients. By the way, that cat lived to be 18 years old, which is pretty good considering his history of illness.

Based on this experience with healing my cat, I thought perhaps there is a cure for breast cancer found with natural substances and prevention. Breast cancer prevention books abound, but except by searching online, I could hardly find any place where prevention of estrogen intake is mentioned as a tool. Why? I don't know! Over 75% of breast cancer is caused by estrogen increase!

Compared to animals, it is a much greater effort for us humans to control our food intake and our environment. We are surrounded by processed foods at the grocery store and are influenced what to eat while at others homes or events. Some of these foods are just plain addictive! Chemicals surround us in our environment that we may be unaware of daily.

Not surprisingly, we have become dependent on modern medicine to resolve illness, however, the recommendations from our doctors and pharmaceutical companies for use of medications many times negate the use of alternative, natural remedies, even if research may support them. There are also viable concerns, regarding the safety and efficacy of natural supplements. Generally, pharmaceutical companies pay to research products that can be patented, so natural remedies are not commonly studied by these companies because they are not easily patented. Occasionally, pharmaceutical companies will take a component of a natural ingredient and separate it out in order to patent it. There are also cases where pharmaceutical companies have used natural products, then patent the delivery method so they can market it. A few of these products are mentioned in Step P.

Studies that are accepted among scientists for cures or solutions are typically *double-blind* (meaning both the patient and researcher don't know what the subject is getting until the end of the study) and *placebo-controlled* (meaning there is a group that receives no treatment, but don't know). Fortunately, these types of studies have been performed on some supplements. You can find the studies on www.pubmed.gov! These are the types of studies that I researched for evidence to support the supplements in Step S.

Researchers and doctors are taking steps to increase the safety of natural remedies. Doctors Catherine Ulbricht, and Ethan Basch, co-founded the Natural Standard Research Collaboration where researchers study all aspects of supplements. Supplements are given grades that reflect the level of available scientific data for or against the use of each therapy for a specific medical condition. Unfortunately, this information is not free for all to use. You would have to pay an annual fee as a researcher or doctor. Some excerpts from their website (www.naturalstandard.com) can be found online. These evaluations are extremely helpful in determining if a supplement may be useful to resolve an illness, if it is potentially harmful or has interactions with other medications. I was able to utilize some of this information for step S.

In addition to utilizing information from www.naturalstandard.com, I researched pubmed.gov, which is a US federal government website that publishes any government funded research on all pharmaceuticals and supplements. I also utilized information on many other websites listed in the resource section, articles and books to point me to research performed on these supplements.

Supplement Use for Prevention

The Mayo Clinic Breast Cancer Book has two chapters devoted to prevention. The authors found that vitamin D, folate, and exercise were negatively correlated with breast cancer. At the same time, they found that alcohol and obesity were positively correlated with breast cancer, both conclusions naturopathic doctors have also reached based on studies. There just might be a few areas of agreement among the medical and natural community!

So, *can* using supplements for prevention be a cure? A supplement is not always adding to something as the name implies. A supplement can actually be removing something from your body. If more people knew the causes of breast cancer and took steps to remove excess estrogen, cases of breast cancer would significantly decrease. Even if people took one step such as having their vitamin D levels checked, at least 50% of breast cancer could be avoided! So yes, supplements can be used toward prevention which ultimately could significantly decrease the amount of breast cancer across our society. Though these steps have not yet been proven to shrink tumors fast enough after breast cancer has already been detected in the individual, they certainly can be a preventative resolution worldwide.

We are battling a war against estrogenic factors. Battle Step S is where we provide the body with some elements it can utilize to get rid of excess estrogen and estrogen-like factors to stop cancer in its tracks. Typically, you would start this step after the next three steps, so read through the end of the S.L.E.E.P. Method before starting any supplement program.

There are so many supplements on the market- it can be overwhelming! The supplements I have selected are those that have scientific evidence to support their use. These are also supplements that I have used. There are additional supplements you can take to flush the body of excess estrogen, which are included the appendix in case you want to review them. I found some of these supplements to be helpful, but others do not have enough research to support them, or have well-known bad side effects.

I have kept Step S as simple and science-based as possible. I have reviewed studies based on the criteria that they have been checked for: safety, effectiveness on cells (in vitro) and animals, and effectiveness on humans. If we are going to be using supplements for prevention, the last thing we want is to take a pill that may not be effective or safe.

I was surprised to find that there are a few cases where natural supplements have actually been approved by the FDA for certain medical uses for prevention. In fact, two of the supplements in this section are approved by the Federal Drug Administration (FDA). The FDA is what gives recommendations for daily allowances for vitamins or supplements (Reference Daily Intake, RDI). Health practitioners do not always agree on these amounts, but I point this out where is applies.

There are seven key supplements with science that supports them. Six are pills and one is a topical liquid. Don't worry! You may only need to take a few of these seven supplements. Some are cancer protective and others are for estrogen detoxification. You can test to see if you even need two of these, vitamin D and iodine. Both can be tested via blood and urine tests respectively. The healthier you are today, the fewer supplements you will need to take. Most people are low in both, however.

Estrogen detoxification is the most important part of this process. I had a friend who was taking cancer protective supplements, but none of the estrogen detox supplements and her thermograms were not improving. Once she started the estrogen detox, thermograms were much better! The doses for estrogen detox supplements are based on having a hormone test result that indicates high estrogen. It only takes one minute per day to take a few pills, so it is worth it. I was on detox supplements for about two years, but I still take Vitamin D as those tests remain in the low range.

Duration of taking supplements can vary. Not all of the supplements will need to be taken indefinitely. Some people may need to take estrogen detox supplements for up to two years, depending on their personal exposure. Tests and symptoms can be used as indicators of when estrogen levels have normalized. A chemist named Roger Mason, recommends not taking any herbal supplement for more than one year as they are not found in our bodies naturally or in common foods in these high doses. Also, most experiments do not test patients for more than one year (although some do). Seek the advice of a doctor for use, especially long-term use of over one year.

Interactions of these supplements with medications has not been checked by me. If you are on any medication, you will want to check with your doctor, pharmacist, *Natural Standard* or *Poison Control*, a free telephone service, to help you find out if there are interactions. First, I'll start with the three supplements that can protect against cancer growth followed by the estrogen detoxification supplements.

Cancer Protective Supplements

Supplement 1: VITAMIN D3

Quantity: 1000 to 5000 IU daily or sun exposure

The medical and alternative community agree that Vitamin D can help prevent breast cancer by as much as 77%.[206] In the last five years, there were over 500 studies on Vitamin D and breast cancer, with many of those being clinical trials. A majority of these studies show a positive effect with sun exposure, high D blood levels and reduced risk of cancers as well as other diseases. There is a reason why there are so many studies going on right now on Vitamin D!

Vitamin D is a powerhouse vitamin. It influences about 10% of all your genes. It up-regulates your ability to fight infections and chronic inflammation. It produces over 200 anti-microbial peptides, one of which is cathelicidin, a broad-spectrum antibiotic. Most importantly, for the purposes of the S.L.E.E.P. Method, it has a number of anticancer effects. One of those is the promotion of cancer cell death. Many studies show that Vitamin D is a potent inhibitor of a cells ability to divide. "Vitamin D metabolites increase communication between cells by switching on a protein that blocks aggressive cell division" says Dr. Cedric Garland, DRPH.[207]

Lastly, vitamin D inhibits the growth of blood vessels that feed a tumor. This is the reason why those people with higher vitamin D blood levels have lower cancer rates. D keeps the tumor from growing in the first place! It also helps breast cells to become more mature, so they are less vulnerable to cancer causing chemicals.

---

[206] Lappe J et al. Jun 2007 *Am J Clin Nutr* "Vitamin D and calcium supplementation reduces cancer risk: results of a randomized trial".
[207] www.nutraceuticalsworld.com Nov 2014 "Vitamin D Linked to Survival of Breast Cancer Patients".

As we grow older, Vitamin D becomes very important because it helps keeps bones stronger as it helps carry calcium to bones. Vitamin D may also decrease estradiol levels, according to a 2010 study.[208] In 2012, scientists actually revealed mechanisms by which vitamin D is effective against estrogen receptor-positive breast cancer cells.[209]

Sunlight is the best way to get vitamin D. Our skin synthesizes vitamin D3 sulfate from sunshine. This is a water-soluble form of vitamin D3 which can travel freely in our bloodstream. Supplemental vitamin D3 is not water soluble and needs cholesterol to transport it (a reason why cholesterol is lowered when supplementing with vitamin D3).

When we lay out in the summer sun mid-day for just a few minutes, our body processes up to 25,000 IU of Vitamin D. So, gaining access to sunlight for 10 to 15 minutes two times per week, without sunscreen should be an adequate amount of Vitamin D for the week. There is even a phone app that you can use called DMinder (dminder.info). It assesses how much UV radiation you are getting and how many IUs of vitamin D your making based on your local weather, skin tone and age. It will also tell you when to get out of the sun to avoid sun burn. If sitting in the sun is not an option, safe tanning beds are. You want to choose a bed with electronic ballasts. These beds do not put out harmful radiation like magnetic ballasts do.

The fact is, most of us do not get enough sun, have access to a safe tanning bed, or have the time to raise our D blood levels naturally. I know I don't! This is why so many of us are deficient in Vitamin D.

Many medical experts are regularly recommending 1000 IU daily for general health. There is no reason to wait for other studies to be completed to decide to raise your vitamin D to optimal levels. Vitamin

---

[208] Knight JA, et al. Mar 2010 *Cancer Causes Control* "Vitamin D association with estradiol and progesterone in young women" This study demonstrated that high vitamin D doses may decrease progesterone and estradiol levels by 3% to 10%.
[209] Krishnan AV et al. Sep 2012 *Steroids* "The potential therapeutic benefits of vitamin D in the treatment of estrogen receptor positive breast cancer".

D has been proven to be completely safe, even at high doses and a safe dose has already been established.

The National Institutes of Health recommends taking 600 IU daily if you are under age 70, and 800 IU daily if over age 70. In 2014, Dr. Cedric Garland and his team at the University of California did a statistical analysis of five studies that showed blood levels of 50 ng/ml is associated with 50% lower risk of death from breast cancer. It also showed that those that consume 4000 IU per day from food or supplement would normally reach a blood level of 50 ng/ml. This study researched 4443 breast cancer patients over nine years.[210]

In the same year, Dr. Garland and team also discovered that in order to achieve protective levels, you have to take much more supplemental vitamin D than previously thought. Study participants had to take 1000 IU to 8000 IU per day to achieve 40 ng/ml blood. This study also concluded that intake of up to 40,000 IUs per day is unlikely to result in vitamin D toxicity (200 ng/mL). Seeing that some of these participants had to take up to 8000 IU daily, it is important that you get your blood tested so you know what dose is right for you! [211]

During seasons of limited sunlight, you may need to take doses on the upper limits. I personally take 1000 IU in summer and 5000 IU in winter. I recently had my D blood levels checked and they were on the low side of normal. This testing helps me gauge how much more vitamin D I may need to take. The blood test is called 25(OH) D or 25-hydroxyvitamin D. Any doctor can give you the lab request for this. You can also order one online at www.grassrootshealth.net for around $70 at the time of this writing.

The normal test result range is 50-70 ng/ml. The result range recommended for people being treated for cancer is 70-100 ng/ml.

---

[210] Mohr SB et al. Mar 2014 *Anticancer Res* "Meta-analysis of vitamin D sufficiency for improving survival of patients with breast cancer".

[211] Garland DF, French CB et al. Feb 2011 *Anticancer Res* "Vitamin D supplement doses and serum 25-hydroxyvitamin D in the range associated with cancer prevention".

Although the lab results may show the normal low range is 30 ng/ml, this is based on the population average, most of which do not have healthy levels. This is one reason Dr. Joseph Mercola and others state levels should be 50 ng/ml or higher.

The other reason is because researchers from the University of San Diego found that low serum vitamin D levels in the months preceding breast cancer diagnosis may predict a high risk of pre-menopausal breast cancer. 1200 healthy women blood levels were studied. Those with low levels of vitamin D had approximately three times the risk of breast cancer as women in the highest vitamin D group. Researchers concluded that women with vitamin D blood serum levels of 50ng/ml or higher reduced their risk by 50%. Breast cancer patients in the US average 17 ng/ml in their blood. Boy, that's low![212]

It is important to note if you are supplementing with high doses of vitamin D3, that you will want to take vitamin K2 as well. This vitamin helps process calcium to the correct places. Otherwise you may get calcium deposits in your kidneys (kidney stones) or worse, arteries. Together, these two vitamins will strengthen your bones and teeth. Some supplement companies are starting to offer one pill with both D3 and K2.

---

[212] www.nutraceuticalsworld.com Nov 2014 "Vitamin D Linked to Survival of Breast Cancer Patients".

Supplement 2: LUGOLS IODINE SPRAY or DROPS

Quantity: Three to five sprays or drops on each breast.

Iodine is a chemical element found in the earth's oceans. Primarily, iodine is needed in the glandular system. The highest concentration of iodine is contained in the thyroid (as iodide). Large amounts are also stored in other areas of the body including the brain, ovaries and the breasts (as iodine).

The breasts need iodine, not iodide. Since iodine is not very soluble in water, it is typically mixed with potassium iodide to increase its solubility. It is also difficult for the stomach to digest iodine, so it can be dissolved in a grain alcohol and sprayed directly on the breast where it can be absorbed through the skin. Each spray of Lugols Iodine has 0.2mg of iodine. This ensures that the iodine will go straight to the breast fat cells. This supplement is *not* a pill, thankfully. But it can be if you prefer it!

The World Health Organization says two billion people suffer from iodine deficiency. According to Dr. David Brownstein, 96% of us are deficient in iodine. Our deficiency exists for several reasons, but the main idea is that iodine, bromine, chloride, and fluoride (all halides on the periodic table) compete with one another for absorption into our cells.

These competing elements are in many items that we ingest every day. Fluoride, which is put into our drinking water and toothpaste, compete with iodine. Chlorine, commonly added to our water, competes with iodine. In addition, iodine is no longer added to salt or bread. It was originally added to bread and salt to prevent swelling of the thyroid (goiter). Iodine has been replaced by bromine in bread and is a toxic substance that has no use for our bodies. Additionally, most iodine has been washed away by rain water from inland areas or is reduced in vegetable crops due to modern farming techniques. We are getting too much fluoride, chlorine and bromide and not enough iodine!

There are over 1100 clinical trials listed on www.pubmed.org about iodine and cancer. There is no scientific evidence that you can overdose on iodine. However, there are case studies where people cannot process iodine effectively or have side effects while taking it. A miniscule percentage of people (.05%) when given 5000mg iodine (a very high dose that is not recommended by any doctors) got hyperthyroid. In most cases, unused iodine is excreted out of the urine. Regardless, using a spray will eliminate any possible side effects.

The RDA of iodine is from 150ug/day to 290ug/day. This amount is enough to prevent an enlarged thyroid but not sufficient for our breast tissue and the rest of the body. Dr. David Brownstein has written several of best-selling books on iodine. He recommends 12.5mg daily for three months.

You can easily test if you are lacking in iodine by spraying some on your breast. If it absorbs quickly, you may be lacking iodine. If it does not absorb within 24 hours, you are most likely not lacking iodine. I tried spraying iodine on my arm and it does not have the same absorption as the breast. My breasts drank it up like lemonade on a hot summer day, my arm, did not have the same effect.

Iodine solution can stain clothes and towels so you will need to let it dry before getting dressed. Also, it turns black if you mix it with baking soda. Since I use baking soda based deodorant, I apply the spray first, let it dry, and then put the deodorant on.

Guess what else iodine is linked to? Maybe you guessed it...estrogen. Scientific studies on animal breast tissue from the 1970s show that iodine deficiency, coupled with proestros from diet or drugs, will show signs of developing breast cancer.[213] [214] Conversely, giving iodine will

---

[213] Eskin BA et al. Jul 1995 *Biol Tr Elem Res* "Different tissue responses for iodine and

suppress breast cancer in animals. Dr. Bernard Eskin, a pioneer researcher, found that when breast cells have blocked access to iodine, it results in precancerous changes that are aggravated when exposed to estrogens or thyroid hormones. When the body is iodine deficient, the breast and the thyroid gland enlarge to compensate for the deficiency. [215] The increased cell growth eventually sets the stage for breast or thyroid cancer.

Iodine also raises your levels of estriol, the good estrogen. According to Doctors Jonathan Wright, Lane Lenard and Dr. David Brownstein, it lowers your own secretion of estrone and estradiol and raises the good estriol. Perhaps this is the reason that Japanese women who have a high intake of iodine containing seafood have lower breast cancer risks. The amount of estriol you have in your body can determine your breast cancer risk. Studies show that low levels of estriol means you have a higher risk. A study performed by the US Army Medical Research and Material Command on 438 pregnant women over the course of 40 years after their pregnancies, found that those in the upper quarter of estriol secretion during pregnancy had a 58 to 77% lower risk of breast cancer than women with the lowest quartile. [216]

Following in the footsteps of Dr. John Meyers of Baltimore, M.D., who originated iodine therapy for fibrocystic breast disease, Dr. David Brownstein worked with over 100 women in his clinic using iodine. Every single woman treated had complete relief of pain of fibrocystic breasts by using iodine within a few weeks to three months. These are pretty amazing results! As a side, a colleague of mine tried iodine for pain with fibrocystic breasts and she did not have positive results using

iodide in rat thyroid and mammary glands".

[214]García-Solís P et al. May 2005 *Mol Cell Endocrinol* "Inhibition of N-Methyl-N-nitrosourea-induced mammary carcinogenesis by molecular iodine (I2) but not by iodide (I-) treatment Evidence that I2 prevents cancer promotion".

[215] Stoddard FR 2nd et al Jul 2008 *Int J Med Sci* "Iodine alters gene expression in the MCF7 breast cancer cell line: evidence for an anti-estrogen effect of iodine".

[216] Siiteri PK et al. 2002 *Department of Defense Breast Cancer Research Meeting* "Prospective study of estrogens during pregnancy and risk of breast cancer."

158

iodine. This just goes to show; there is not one thing that works for everyone.

Not only does iodine do great things with your estrogen levels, it has been shown to actually kill off cancer cells. Only Mexico and India have done recent studies on this; Mexico in 2005 and India in 2006. Two studies in India found that iodine kills cancer cells but not normal cells. The breast cancer cells killed off included MCF-7, MDA-MB-231, MDA-MB-453, 2R75-1 and T-47D.[217] [218] From these studies, we can see that adding iodine not only can help prevent breast cancer, it can also help treat it! Since iodine is not patentable, not much has been done in terms of research more recently.

Iodine is the safest among all the elements. Not only can the right dose prevent breast cancer, it can give you energy and has been known to actually cure thyroid disorders. As far back as 1996 in the *Journal of Clinical Endocrinology,* scientists showed a relationship with breast cancer and hypothyroid. Just maybe we are all just too low in iodine.[219]

I did an iodine urine challenge test to check my iodine levels before using the supplement form of iodine. I have had hypothyroid since 2002 and tested low. My results showed 38% iodine, which is low (90% excretion is normal). Kits are available online. I ordered mine from Hakala Research Laboratory. Hakala is one of the recommended labs by Dr. David Brownstein, and has the benefit of being more affordable than other similar options.

Additionally, you can test for other competing halides of iodine such as bromine and fluoride. I tested bromine along with the iodine test and

[217] Shrivastava A et al. Jul 2006 *J Biol Chem* "Molecular iodine induces caspase-independent apoptosis in human breast carcinoma cells involving the mitochondria-mediated pathway".
[218] Singh P et al. Nov 2011 *Biochem Biophys Res Commun* "Inhibition of autophagy stimulate molecular iodine-induced apoptosis in hormone independent breast tumors".
[219] Giani C et al. Mar 1996 *J Clin Endocrinol Metab* "Relationship between breast cancer and thyroid disease: relevance of autoimmune thyroid disorders in breast malignancy."

tested low in bromine; thank goodness. I decided to add the pill form, *Iodoral* to my supplement list instead of doing the topical spray. Both Dr. Brownstein and Dr. Bruce Rind recommend starting with ½ tablet daily. My side effects were minimal at this dose.

Unfortunately, I am included in a small percentage of people who have weird side effects. While taking iodine, I had to slowly titer the dose up as the effects subsided. My side effects included acne at first, heart palpitations, fatigue and weird dreams. After three months on iodine, I was able to reduce my hypothyroid medication (Levothyroxine) and completely stop one other medication (Armour Thyroid)! My iodine test results came back almost normal at 80% at the end of these three months.

I later did another test and found out I have a problem transporting iodine into my thyroid. While this result is beyond the scope of this book, it is important to note that working with a doctor while supplementing with high dose iodine pills (above 290 ug/day), is imperative. The iodine can cause you to get better (in 35% of patients) or have temporary toxin release side effects. If you have hypothyroid and are on medication, have high blood pressure or are sensitive to supplements and medications, *Lugols* Spray is the way to go.

As an aside, there is another form of iodine called nascent iodine. This is a liquid form that tastes better than Lugol's solution and is supposedly easier to absorb (bio available) into your system. Dr. Mark Sircus posts that this form of iodine's side effects are less compared to those of *Iodoral* and dosing can be done throughout the day.[220] Since there is more scientific data about dosing with *Iodoral* and no studies listed on www.pubmed.gov on nascent iodine, I chose *Iodoral*.

Supplement 3: CURCUMIN

Quantity: One 600 mg capsule per day or two, 250mg capsules per day

---

[220] http://drsircus.com/medicine/iodine/iodine-dosages

Curcumin was not originally recommended to me for preventing breast cancer, but due to overwhelming scientific evidence and its current use alongside modern medicine, I have included it.

Curcumin is one of three components in the spice turmeric. *Curcuma longa* is a ginger like plant that grows in tropical regions. The roots of the plant contain turmeric and curcumin. Curcumin has been used in medicine for centuries. It has over ten ways to block cancer in general. It is not well absorbed as a spice but better as a supplement says Joe Pizzorno, N.D. author of *Natural Medicine for the Prevention and Treatment of Cancer* (Riverhead Trade).

Specific to breast cancer, curcumin does several things. First, it blocks many proestros from getting inside cells. These proestros can be man-made like pesticides like DDT, dioxin, Chlordane, endosulfane, and paraquat (weed killer). They can also be nitrosamines (in cooked lunch meats), carbon tetrachloride (a solvent in varnish), or chemicals that contaminate America's water and food. It actually blocks these chemicals from getting inside the cells.[221] We can think of curcumin as our amour amidst a world of attackers.

Not only does curcumin prevent proestros from getting inside cells, it blocks grow signals from reaching cells. It blocks multiple kinds of kinases (substances that allow enzyme changes), one of which is called PKC or protein kinase C and another called PI3K/AKT. Studies show that curcumin significantly slows the growth of any cancer that uses PKC or PI3K/AKT to grow, one of which is breast cancer but includes glioma (brain or spine), prostate, skin and lung cancers.

Pharmaceutical companies have made drugs such as *Yervoy* that model the inhibitory effect curcumin has on kinases. In fact, curcumin blocks CTLA-4, a protein receptor found on immune system cells, that prevents the immune system from attacking cancer just as *Yervoy* does.

---

[221] Jul 2002 *Life Extension Magazine* "A Report on Curcumin's Anti-Cancer Effects"

[222] [223] *Yervoy* is a drug that received FDA approval in 2011. There have been hundreds of animal trials showing curcumin prevents or shrinks tumors in the colon, skin, stomach, liver, lung, and breast. There are numerous studies on human breast cancer cells also showing curcumin's effectiveness against cancer cells.[224] [225] Human case studies and placebo controlled studies are limited, but some show problems with absorption of the spice. Ongoing studies are being performed, but many people today are using it.

Thirdly, curcumin reactivates a tumor suppressor gene in breast cancer cells known as the RASSF1-A gene.[226] There are at least five other great things that curcumin does in regards to cancer such as reduce inflammation, protect against radiation, enhance immunity, and stop angiogenesis (the secretion of substances that causes cancer cell blood vessels to grow), but the one that caught my attention most was that it actually killed cancer cells in the G2 stage of growth. Curcumin has demonstrated this with human leukemia cells, lung, prostate, and thyroid cancerous cells and now in ras and HER2 breast cancer gene cells.[224] For this reason, cancer patients are using curcumin to kill off cancer cells. Why don't we hear about this?

Another interesting fact: did you know that cancer patients are given curcumin by their doctors to alleviate symptoms from chemotherapy? The dose cancer patients take is usually between 1800 to 3600 mg per day. Its safety has been proven and it is being used regularly! We can

---

[222] Sharma S et al. Jan 2007 *Clin Exp Immunol* "Resveratrol and curcumin suppress immune response through CD28/CTLA-4 and CD80 co-stimulatory pathway".

[223] Stanberry, Porter Oct 2014 *"The Next Big Step Forward for Cancer Treatment"*.

[224] Catania A et al. Aug 2013 *Breast Cancer Res Treat* "Immunoliposome encapsulation increases cytotoxic activity and selectivity of curcumin and resveratrol against HER2 overexpressing human breast cancer cells".

[225] Chen WC et al. Dec 2013 *J Agric Food Chem* "Curcumin suppresses doxorubicin-induced epithelial-mesenchymal transition via the inhibition of TGF-β and PI3K/AKT signaling pathways in triple-negative breast cancer cells".

[226] Du L et al. 2012 *Nutr Cancer* "Reactivation of RASSF1A in breast cancer cells by curcumin".

wait for all the official human studies, but the ruling is already out. Curcumin is generally safe, and can help deter cancer.

It is important to note that curcumin can interfere with some chemotherapy drugs, such as *Camptosar* (irinotecan). Also, high doses of "thiol" nutrients such as cysteine, lipoic acid, SAMe and glutathione may interfere with its ability to inhibit PKC in actively growing cancer. Additionally, there are conflicting studies about taking it with Herceptin. It was not recommended in one article while taking Herceptin or having an inflammatory issue, but the cellular study in 2013 showed that Herceptin actually increased the efficacy of curcumin and resveratrol.[224] Therefore, if you currently are diagnosed with breast cancer and HER2 positive, check with your doctor before supplementing with curcumin.

I used curcumin to treat my chronic Lyme disease (another good healing story for another time). I had side effects (Lyme bacteria die-off reactions) at the 600-mg dose. If you have, or suspect you have Lyme disease, you may want to consider a lower dose (100 mg per day) to start out and then titer up to 500 or 600 mg per day. For those with Lyme disease, it is also a good idea to pulse curcumin at monthly intervals. Go to a higher dose (1200mg) for one or two months, then take a break for one month. This allows the bacteria to come out from hiding and then be killed off some more when you re-introduce curcumin. Ha, ha we can trick those little buggers!

It is important to buy the right kind of curcumin. As mentioned previously, there have been studies that report it is not highly absorbable in the stomach (bioavailable). Ways to avoid this are to stay away from any additives that affect bioavailability. A few of these are listed at the end of this section. Also, you can use the spice turmeric on your food to get some curcumin without taking a pill, although it is not as effective as in high dose supplements.

To recap the three cancer protective supplements listed here, vitamin D blocks cancer growth, iodine suppresses cancer growth through hormonal pathways and actually kills cancer cells and curcumin kills cancer cells in the G2 stage! Boom! Those three supplements alone are amazing for breast cancer prevention!

Estrogen Detoxification Supplements

Supplement 4: DIM (Diindolylmethane)

Quantity: Take one or two 100 mg caps per day.

DIM, also known as Diindolylmethane, makes healthier estrogens. Specifically, it makes 2-hydroxyestrone, one of the good estrogens and is a natural anti-carcinogen. You can think of DIM as just eating a bunch of cruciferous vegetables (broccoli, cabbage, Brussels sprouts etc.) in pill form, so no harm done. Your DIM supplement should be combined with Vitamin E TPGS (Tocophersolan) for better absorption. Vitamin E TPGS is so safe, it appears on the "Generally Regarded as Safe" (GRAS) list published by the FDA. It is also recommended by the Breast Cancer Prevention Institute in its online *Breast Cancer Risks and Prevention* booklet.

Diindolylmethane is a compound resulting from digestion of cruciferous vegetables. According to the NIH National Cancer Institute, DIM is a phytonutrient and plant indole found in cruciferous vegetables including broccoli, Brussels sprouts, cabbage, cauliflower and kale, with potential anti-androgenic and anti-neoplastic activities. A 2013 scientific review showed thirteen studies proving high cruciferous vegetable consumption is directly associated with a reduced risk of breast cancer.[227] One study performed in 2001 published by the *Journal of American Medical Association* demonstrated that women who ate 1.5 servings of broccoli daily, had a 42% lower cancer risk.[228]

---

[227] Liu X and Lv K June 2013 *Breast* "Cruciferous vegetables intake is inversely associated with risk of breast cancer: a meta-analysis".

[228] Terry P et al. June 2001 *Journal of American Medical Association* "Brassica vegetables and breast cancer risk".

NIH says the phytochemical in broccoli that has anticancer activity against estrogens is I3C (Indole-3-Carbinole). These I3Cs form DIM which in turn naturally produce 2-hydroxestrone, a healthy estrogen. 2-hydroxestrone naturally deters production of 16-hydroxyestrone, one of the proestros that causes breast cancer cell growth. Many studies demonstrate this.[229] Per Doctor Jonathan Wright's book, one research report found that I3C also lowers 4-hydroxyestrogen (another proestro), so it is very likely that DIM does the same.

Michael A. Zeligs, M.D. has identified DIM as the safest, most active and most beneficial I3C-related substance found in cruciferous vegetables. A study published in 2008 showed there were no side effects up to 300mg doses in humans.[230]

In addition to increasing good estrogen, DIM prevents cancer growth in other ways. Research in 2009 at the University of California, showed that DIM reduces the production of two proteins (CXCR4 and CXCL12) needed for breast and ovarian cancer to spread.[231] According to NIH, DIM also induces apoptosis (cell death) in tumor cells. Basically, an agent that induces apoptosis in tumor cells is capable of killing off cancer cells. Hey NIH, I think that is pretty good!

According to my research, there are approximately 75 studies published on DIM regarding breast and cervical cancer. Many of these studies have been performed in cells or on mice. There are also several studies on humans that date as far back as 1991. Because of the great results with these studies, ongoing placebo controlled human testing has been and is being performed. All tests are confirming DIM's benefit

---

[229] Michnovicz JJ and Bradlow HL 1991 *Nutr Cancer* "Altered estrogen metabolism and excretion in humans following consumption of indole-3-carbinol."

[230] Reed GA et al. Oct 2008 *Cancer Epidemiol Biomarkers Prev* "Single-dose pharmacokinetics and tolerability of absorption-enhanced 3, 3''diindolylmethane in healthy subjects."

[231] Hsu EL et al. Mar 2009 *J Oncol* University of California, Los Angeles "Modulation of CXCR4, CXCL12, and Tumor Cell Invasion Potential in Vitro by Phytochemicals."

for breast, prostate, ovarian and cervical cancer risk reduction. DIM is one supplement you cannot go without if you are trying to get the proestros out or lower estrogen levels! (See Appendix A for additional studies on a DIM all-in-one supplement called *BreastDefend®*)

Supplement 5: TRIMETHYGLYCINE (TMG)

Quantity: one 750 mg cap once or twice daily without food.

TMG is an amino acid also known as betaine and dimethylglycine. TMG is found in a variety of plant (most notably beets) and animal sources and aids in several chemical processes. TMG is actually made in our bodies, but most people do not make enough of it. According to Dr. Lawrence Wilson, the reason appears to be the presence of heavy metals, stress, infections, disease or inflammation, which use up TMG. Even if you try to eat plenty of vegetables, your body still may not get enough TMG.

TMG has three methyl groups joined to one molecule of glycine. When TMG is present, it easily lets go of two or even three of its methyl groups, which frees up dimethylglycine or glycine to be utilized elsewhere in the body. When giving up TMG's methyl groups, your body may be left with dimethylglycine (DMG).

DMG is considered a B-complex vitamin which can help with stress and improve liver activity and athletic performance, among other things. More importantly, DMG has anti-inflammatory effects, improves immunity, shrinks tumors and enhances anti-tumor defenses.

A study published in 2012 reported the anti-angiogenic action of betaine.[232] Angiogenesis causes cancerous blood vessels to grow. Betaine inhibited angiogenesis and decreased tissue cell growth factors. The process of angiogenesis is an important step for tumor

---

[232] Yi EY, Kim YJ Nov 2012 *Int J Oncol* "Betaine inhibits in vitro and in vivo angiogenesis through suppression of the NF-κB and Akt signaling pathways".

growth and metastasis, as is inflammation. Betaine is known to suppress inflammation as well. [233] For this reason, angiogenesis inhibitors that also suppress inflammation have been studied for anticancer treatment.

In regards to hormones, chemicals and heavy metals, TMG supports the exit pathway that excess by-products take to get out of the body. TMG helps this pathway by breaking down toxic estrogens into friendly ones and neutralizing toxic properties. It does this by making the chemicals more water soluble. TMG also raises 2ME2 levels. This acts as anti-carcinogenic protection against hormone induced cancers such as breast, ovary and prostate.

This is what www.anabolicmen.com says about betaine for its use in their three-part estrogen flush recommendation:

"By design your estrogen molecules are all missing one methyl group, and this means that your liver can't chelate them out of the body. In other words, they're stuck inside of you...

...And this is where methylators get involved. Because when you consume a methylator (choline or betaine) you introduce those missing methyl groups into the body. The methyl groups will then "complete" the empty spots in the estrogen molecules, which makes it possible for your liver to chelate them out of the body.

Another process TMG helps with is the reduction of homocysteine.[234] Its methyl group donation is used in the conversion of homocysteine to methionine. If you have a high level of homocysteine in your blood, it makes you prone to cell injury, which leads to inflammation in the blood vessels. This in turn may make you prone to heart disease due to

[233] Olli K et al. Jan 2013 *Br J Nutr* "Betaine reduces the expression of inflammatory adipokines caused by hypoxia in human adipocytes".

[234] Olthof MR et al. 2003 *J Nutr* "Low dose betaine supplementation leads to immediate and long term lowering of plasma homocysteine in healthy men and women."

blockage of blood flow. High homocysteine is associated with breast cancer as well.[235] TMG is FDA approved for reducing homocysteine levels and is safe.[236]

There is yet another process that TMG is involved in. It has the ability to stimulate production of S-Adenosylmethionine (SAMe). Again, TMG has three methyl groups. These methyl groups are added to homocysteine, which are eventually converted to SAMe. SAMe protects the liver and is a natural antidepressant. SAMe then acts as a methyl donor for DNA. Methyl groups are needed when our cells make copies of DNA to RNA. Genetic copy errors can occur without enough TMG. When methyl groups are attached to DNA, they are protective in that they prevent mutating genes from expressing themselves. Here is how you can help protect your genes from making photo copies of errors and keep any defective genes at bay! Animal studies show that TMG may be a preventer of cancer due to this DNA protection. Sex drive can also be increased by SAMe due to increased dopamine levels.

The most noticeable effect of TMG for me was increased energy. It may have helped with sex drive too, but various other hormonal factors could have been at play here. Overall, TMG reduces coronary heart failure risk by reducing inflammation, improves cognitive function, reduces the risk of genetically induced cancers, slows cellular aging, increases SAMe and decreases toxic estrogens and chemicals. Doesn't it sound like a good idea to take some TMG? It has been shown to be safe if taken orally up to 3 grams twice per day. Dr. Lawrence Wilson gives doses of 1000 to 3000mg per day with no side effects, except in rare cases.

---

[235] Akilzhanova A et al. Sep 2013 *Anticancer Res* "Genetic profile and determinants of homocysteine levels in Kazakhstan patients with breast cancer"

[236] Schwab U, Torronen A et al. 2005 J Nutr "Orally administered betaine has an acute and dose-dependent effect on serum betaine and plasma homocysteine concentrations in healthy humans".

Supplement 6: CALCIUM-D-GLUCARATE

Quantity: Take one to two 500mg capsules two to three times per day, depending on total elevated estrogens.

Calcium-D-Glucarate (CDG) is a natural substance that is produced in small amounts in humans but is also found in highest amounts in apples, oranges, broccoli, spinach and Brussels sprouts. Taking high amounts of CDG has shown to inhibit beta-glucuronidase, an enzyme produced in the colon that is involved in Phase II liver detoxification. [237] Elevated levels of beta-glucuronidase has been associated with hormone-dependent cancers such as breast cancer. [238] [239] Inhibition of this enzyme, therefore, decreases the risk of breast cancer. [240] [241] CDG helps maintain the bond that is formed between toxic estrogens and glucuronic acid in the liver so that it can be carried out of the body and not re-circulated. Basically, CDG helps get the estrogen molecules to exit the body and not re-absorb. [242]

There is not enough CDG in food or our bodies to remove stored estrogen. 500 mgs are recommended, but more can be taken without any side effects. This is about equal to 82 pounds of fresh fruit and vegetables! The recommended dose for humans is currently 500 to 4500mg per day depending on how high your estrogen levels are or if you currently have cancer. [243]

---

[237] Walaszek Z et al. 1997 *Cancer Detect Prev* "Metabolism, uptake, and excretion of D-glucaric acid salt and its potential use in cancer prevention."

[238] Heerdt AS et al. 1995 *Isr J Med Sci* "Calcium glucarate as a chemopreventive agent in breast cancer".

[239] Hanausek, M et al. June 2003 *Integr Cancer Ther* "Detoxifying Cancer Causing Agents to Prevent Cancer".

[240] Selkirk JK, Cohen GM, MacLeod MC. 1980 *Arch Toxicol* "Glucuronic acid conjugation in the metabolism of chemical carcinogens by rodent cells."

[241] Abou-Issa H et al. 1995 *Cancer Res* "Relative efficacy of glucarate on the initiation and promotion phases of rat mammary carcinogenesis."

[242] Walaszek Z et al. 1986 *Carcinogenesis* "Dietary glucarate as anti-promoter of 7, 12-dimethylbenz[a]anthracene-induced mammary tumorigenesis." (Reduction of estrogen by 23%)

There are over 80 cellular and animal based laboratory studies on Calcium-D-Glucarate and cancer. Although there are few human clinical trials, ongoing studies show promising results. Preliminary human trials show there are no adverse reactions or toxic effect if taking too much.

According to a couple of online articles, there were clinical trials taking place, initiated by the National Cancer Institute in the 2002 timeframe to determine whether CDG could be as effective as tamoxifen for preventing breast cancer. I was unable to locate these clinical trials online, but I was able to locate a 2003 review which stated that CDG offers a promising cancer prevention approach and may be more effective than tamoxifen.[244] Additionally, many animal study results have been very positive. One study showed CDG was able to reduce the number of estrogen receptors by 48%. In rats, CDG reduced breast cancer by 70%.[245]

For dosing, there are studies that disclose doses rats were given. Typically, rats were given at least 200 mg per 1 kg (2.2 pounds). [246] These are very high amounts compared to what is recommended for humans. There were no adverse effects, but it remains to be proven in human clinical trials that estrogen reducing effects remain at lower doses.

Supplement 7: MILK THISLE or SILYMARIN

Quantity: Take 100 to 400 mg daily.

Milk thistle is a plant that exists all over the world. It produces red to purple flowers. Milk thistle extract is made from its seeds and may have

---

[243] www.bulletproofexec.com/calcium-d-glucarate

[244] Hanausek, M et al. June 2003 *Integr Cancer Ther* "Detoxifying Cancer Causing Agents to Prevent Cancer".

[245] www.bulletproofexec.com/calcium-d-glucarate

[246] Walaszek Z et al. Jan 1990 *Cancer Lett* "Antiproliferative effect of dietary glucarate on the Sprague-Dawley rat mammary gland".

several components, including silymarin, a group of flavonolignans. Silymarin is what effectively detoxes estrogens out and prevents toxin build-up of the liver.

There are many good effects from milk thistle. Milk thistle was once used to help the milk flow in nursing mothers, hence the name. Another good effect from milk thistle is that is strengthens the outer membranes of the liver cells, which prevents poisons and damaging substances from entering the cell. It also reduces inflammation, which can help with many liver problems and the immune system. Third, it increases the flow of bile from the liver and gallbladder, which remove bad estrogens among other things. This is the main reason we are using milk thistle here. It is also known to help and reduce symptoms from cirrhosis, death cap mushroom poisoning, hepatitis and gallstones.

Milk thistle has over 120 published studies on pubmed.gov. Humans have been using it for over 2000 years. Silymarin is the active compound found in the herb milk thistle. It protects the liver from damage. It has been found to be safe and well tolerated. Only high doses above 1500mg/day were found to have mild allergic reactions. [247]

In 2007 *Integrative Cancer Therapies* published a review of several clinical trials involving milk thistle and cancer.[248] The researchers stated that the future of milk thistle for cancer was promising. There have been three case studies where The National Cancer Institute supports the use of milk thistle for a variety of other diseases as well. None of the cancer studies are related to breast cancer.

If we are going to be detoxing bad estrogens out, we need to make sure we do it without harming our body. If the liver is not working properly, we can't pull chemicals out of the tissues. Synthetic and chemical

[247] National Cancer Institute Milk Thistle PDQ 8/10/2012

[248] Greenlee H et al. Jun 2007 *Integr Cancer Ther* "Clinical applications of Silybum marianum in oncology".

hormones are processed by the liver. Protecting and supporting the liver before and during an estrogen detoxification protocol is important. If the liver doesn't process the hormones out, they will be stored as fat and perhaps cause estrogen toxicity. We don't want that!

If you are going to be using iodine in pill form, you may also be detoxing heavy metals during this process. Milk thistle will also effectively process heavy metals through your liver.

Additional Supplements: See Appendix A

Supplement Quality

There are a few important considerations to know about supplementation. If you are going to buy supplements, it would be good to know their quality! If we take into consideration the goal for most companies to make a profit, decisions about ingredients may not always be the best for you. A recent scandal exposed in New York told that supplements were being sold in stores without the actual ingredients in them. In addition to not having the ingredient in the first place, some ingredients may cost less, not be as pure or as bio-available. It is important to know who you are buying your supplements from and which ingredients are considered substandard.

Here is a list of ingredients to watch out for:

- No listing of other ingredients on the label. There are always other ingredients. If there are no other ingredients listed, what are they trying to hide?

- Magnesium stearate listed in other ingredients. This is used as a flowing agent to help get the product into the capsule or mold. It is known to possibly reduce the absorption of the supplement in your digestive system. This will not hurt you, just lower the absorption. Avoid this if possible.

-Polysorbate 80: affects the absorption of the ingredient

-Isopropyl Myrislate: affects the absorption of the ingredient

- Soy: Most soy grown in the US is GMO. Ingesting anything with soy may mean that you are ingesting pesticides by doing so, and possibly increasing estrogen.

- Number of pills: When comparing two different brand names, check the number of pills it takes to get to equal milligrams. Also check the quantity of pills in the bottle. Some might take four pills instead of two. In that case, the bottle will not last as long and you may end up spending a lot more money if you buy the brand with four pills.

Good ingredients to look for:

- Black pepper extract – aids in absorption of supplements.

Through research and several doctor recommendations, I found some of the better quality manufacturers are Thorne Research, Integrative Therapeutics, Allergy Research Group, Innate, Gaia, EcoNugenics, Xymogen and Perque.

Chapter 13

L is for LIFESTYLE CHANGE

Battle Step L is where the mind and body connect. We use our mind to make educated decisions about our lifestyle and put them into actions that affect the body. The good thing about lifestyle change, is there are no bad side effects which means these methods can be used during treatment of breast cancer. The American Institute of Cancer Research determined from a review that up to 40% of all breast cancer cases could be prevented with lifestyle measures such as exercising and maintaining a healthy weight. One thing I found out, is that these two measures directly affect estrogen and how it is stored in the body.

This step is the most important change you can make. As you can see from the risk factor table earlier, there are many lifestyle factors that can increase or decrease your risk of breast cancer. Once you are aware of these, it is up to you to implement the actions that are right for you.

Battle Step L against proestros is about willingly choosing to stop putting patentable hormones into the body and work on eliminating them using the body's internal detoxification process. One of the most important decisions in your life is about whether you will use patentable hormones in the form of birth control and if so, for how long. In addition, taking time out for yourself with meditation, prayer, relaxation and exercise involves prioritizing, making this action difficult. When you succeed, it makes for a balanced life. Carving out a few extra chunks of time for myself, was the most invigorating action I took.

It's all too easy to get lost in a sea of people and commitments that make up our busy lives. Women are generally *givers,* spending money, energy and time on others, sometimes at the expense of their own well-being. It is not selfish to put your mental and physical health first;

being there for your friends and family requires you to replenish yourself and prioritize. If we want to achieve goals while here on this earth, we must be alive and healthy in the first place. The old adage rings true: you don't have anything if you don't have your health!

Change 1: PATENTABLE HORMONE USE

Short-term only and none prior to age 20

Goodbye pills, patches and IUD's! You have seen in the previous chapters and in my own thermograms what patentable hormones can do to breast cancer risk. 17% of us have taken birth control pills that have patentable estrogen or progestins. Some of us have used a hormone IUD; *Mirena, Paraguard or Skyla* and/or the patch. Still others have used the day after pill known at Plan B or taken the abortion pill. These methods all have levonorgestrel in them, a progestin known to be associated with breast cancer. Plan B is equal to ingestion of 40-50 birth control pills at one time (FDA 2013). [249] This is not natural to our body and in some ways our body processes these patentable hormones like an estrogen.

If you decide to do the full S.L.E.E.P. Method, it will be imperative to not use any of these birth control methods prior to starting it. It will have very little effect if you are on these types of birth control. Hey, this is one instance where you actually stop taking a pill! I am not the only one recommending you get off these after four years of use. The Breast Cancer Prevention Institute in their online "Breast Cancer Risks and Prevention" booklet also recommends it. To re-affirm, here are the reasons to stop using patentable hormones:

1. High breast cancer risk: Women who are currently or have recently (past 8 to 10 years) used the birth control pill have a 20 to 104% increased risk for breast cancer. Women who use the Pill after the age

---

[249] Yager J, Davidson N Jan 2006 *N Engl J Med* "Estrogen Carcinogenesis in Breast Cancer".

of 45 have a 144% greater risk of developing breast cancer than women who have never used it. [250] [251]

There are also risks for younger users of birth control. Sam Epstein MD, an author of *The Breast Cancer Prevention Program* book, wrote in 1997 that "more than 20 well-controlled studies have demonstrated the clear risk of premenopausal breast cancer with the use of oral contraceptives". As seen in my relative risk table, this means that young women during their teens or twenties who use oral contraceptives, have 22 to 52% relative risk for developing breast cancer compared to a non-user.

2. Low sex drive: Replacement estrogens elevate SHBG (steroid hormone binding globulin) which in turn lowers androgen levels. These are the hormones that directly affect your sex drive. No wonder I had no sex drive after using the pill all those years!

3. Adds hormones to the water supply if on septic system.

Agreeable Birth Control

What are we supposed to do if we can't use patentable hormones forever? Taking birth control is one of the largest ways we put proestros into our body. We use the pill, patch or uterine device to avoid getting pregnant. Planning or not planning to have children is one of the most important things in a women's life. Many of us would rather be reading *"What to Expect When We're Not Expecting"*! We try our best to get the most effective, 99.9% accurate birth prevention tool.

---

[250] Kahlenborn C et al. 2006 *Mayo Clinic Proceedings* "Oral Contraceptive Use as a Risk Factor for Premenopausal Breast Cancer: A Meta-analysis".

[251] Kahlenborn C. 2000 *One More Soul*, 228-229. "Overall cancer risk from several cancers due to oral contraceptive use: Breast Cancer, Its Link to Abortion and the Birth Control Pill".

I am here to tell you that is going to be okay. There are ways we can still plan without having to use patentable hormones for an extended period.

Typically, there will be many years that we will plan on not having children which is why it would be good to have an alternative form of birth control in mind. Even if you decide to play it safe and use the pill for less than eight years after your first child, eventually you will need some sort of birth control. Unfortunately, there is no 100% method, save abstinence and there is not much on the market that doesn't have some sort of hormone in it.

If we look at the big picture, women these days are looking at 30 plus years of birth control methods if they plan on only having two children. Of course, if you plan on having children early, it is good for breast lobule growth, but for obvious reasons, not everyone has or wants this choice. The next paragraph outlines an example of safer birth control throughout a woman's life.

As a teen or young adult, the condom, diaphragm or family planning methods could be utilized. After having a first child and in between children, the pill, patch or other hormonal method could be used for up to eight years. After having children, the copper IUD could be a consideration for an additional five years, dependent on heavy metal testing and prior hormone use. Near and around menopause, condoms, diaphragms or natural family planning would again be the birth control methods of choice.

I thought it was very interesting and alarming that while I was detoxing my body of estrogens, my body decided it wanted to expel the *Mirena* after having it in for three years. It was literally screaming "get the heck out! I woke up in the middle of the night with excruciating cramps. I have to say, it was even worse than labor, and I did that *au naturel*. I thought I was going to die. I had to wake up my husband and take some ibuprofen. Thank goodness for ibuprofen, because I don't think I could have lived through the night without going to ER. The next day I went to the midwife who had delivered my baby and had her deliver that *Mirena*! Of course, they tested me for diseases and pregnancy, which came back negative. All this happened while I was doing the S.L.E.E.P. Method estrogen detox supplement protocol. This is definitely a good reason to get hormonal IUDs out before starting the detox protocol!

The *Mirena* releases "Levonorgestrel", a second-generation progestin (patentable hormone). You bet your bottom dollar that progestin was the cause of all this trouble. The midwife said that very occasionally this will happen. A person's body will reject the IUD, but it usually happens when it is first inserted. It is obvious to me that my body was trying to detox it right out of me. Needless to say, I had to choose another birth control method. These are the options I was given that have no synthetic hormones.

- The diaphragm with spermicidal
- The male or female condom
- The copper IUD (copper is a proestro, however)
- Spermicidal inserts (Some spermicides are proestros)
- Rhythm Method
- Natural Family Planning (NFP)
- Vasectomy or Sterilization

You can choose a combination of a few of these like the rhythm method, the condom and the diaphragm. To be the most 99.9% effective, I use an *Android* phone application to track fertility cycles. Calculating with a regular calendar is how I got pregnant in the first place! It is critical to use something reliable that will be able to tell you how long your cycles are so you can give or take a few days during ovulation to be extra careful. If you are not regular, using progesterone cream as described later will help regulate your cycle.

During ovulation time, the diaphragm with spermicide and a condom can be used or choose abstinence. This is the time to be the most careful. Unfortunately, spermicides come with parabens and condoms have plastics and other cell promoting ingredients. There are some

178

alternative safer choices out there if you want to be really careful with proestros. During the rest of the month, one method can be used.

Vasectomies and having your tubes tied may not be a really a good idea. Your hormones get all off kilter when you do that. My friend completely lost her sex drive after having her tubes tied and she was only 27 years old. It is very sad. If you do have a hysterectomy (uterine removal), keep your ovaries so you still have your own hormones being produced and won't need to supplement. Also, removal of ovaries has an increase in death due to lung cancer and other diseases associated with it.[252]

There are several natural family planning methods available. They include the Billings Ovulatory Method and NaPro Technology, which is based on the Creighton model (over 30 years of documented scientific research on the menstrual and fertility cycle). These are also used by women to help with infertility. This is one way that fertility drugs can be avoided. As a side note, another way to avoid fertility drugs is to have your hormones tested and utilize bioidentical progesterone cream!

If you need help choosing an alternative birth control method, it may be helpful to read a blog by Katie at www.wellnessmama.com. Her article titled "Natural alternatives to Hormonal Contraceptives" reviews them. Should you decide to utilize the rhythm method and do not have a regular cycle, you will need to monitor your cycles using temperature or other modalities. Katie reviews fertility monitors in her blog "Using Natural Fertility Monitors". She has chosen OvaCue as her method of choice because it has a 98% accuracy rate and has the ability to predict ovulation 7 days in advance. Thank you, Katie, for your helpful reviews!

Of course, using these monitors lets you know when you're fertile so you can abstain from intercourse or use extra precaution like the condom and diaphragm together. As stated before, if you have a fairly

---

[252] Parker WH et al. 2009 *Obstet Gynecol* "Ovarian conservation at the time of hysterectomy and long-term health outcomes in the Nurses' Health Study".

regular cycle, you can chart your cycle on a phone application and it will let you know when your fertile window is. None of the temperature monitoring is really necessary if you are regular. If you are irregular, then temperature monitoring will be crucial. Once you get used to testing, documenting and charting, it really just becomes part of your routine.

Change 2: DE-STRESS

If you find that people often say you need to sit down and relax, that may be a clue that you are stressed. We are often so stressed; we don't even realize it because we don't even know what relaxed feels like. To find out what that feels like, we need to spend some time by ourselves, relaxing. In my house, we allocate this personal time on the calendar.

First, we need to understand that stress is directly linked to high cortisol levels in our bodies, which in turn increases our risk for breast cancer. Cortisol has been proven to have a direct effect on estrogen.[253] Cortisol may alter the generation or activity of estrogen by increasing it! It does this by several known mechanisms. One is by increasing aromatase activity around breast tumors.[254] A second way is by obstructing cell growth control of BRCA1 gene.[255] Thirdly, stress due to life events when young, causes permanent changes in the HPA-axis responsiveness, which affects how the body handles stress in the future.[256]

---

[253] Simpson E, Akerman G et al. 1981 *Proc Natl Acad Sci* USA "Estrogen formation in stromal cells of adipose tissue of women: induction by glucocorticosteroids".

[254] Schmidt M, Loffler G 1994 FEBS Lett "Induction of aromatase in stromal vascular cells from human breast adipose tissue depends on cortisol growth factors."

[255] Antonova L, Mueller C 2008 *Genes, Chromosomes Cancer* "Hydrocortisone down regulates the tumor suppressor gene BRCA1 in mammary cells: a possible molecular link between stress and breast cancer."

[256] Elzinga BM Feb 2008 *Psychoneuroendocrinology* "Diminished cortisol responses to psychosocial stress associated with lifetime adverse events a study among healthy subjects".

We all know stress is not good for the body, but now we know it can actually be part of the proestro problem! It only takes spending ten minutes a day surrounded by no one to have a complete change in stress levels. Getting yourself alone in a room with the door locked is half the battle, especially during life crisis. The other half is mind control. It really is amazing what you can feel when you just do nothing. Those precious minutes can be used for relaxing your body and your mind. Some ways to do this are: meditate, pray, stretch, do yoga, listen to soft music, read, or sit in a sauna/steam bath, or massage chair.

Sometimes, it may be difficult to carve out ten minutes per day so another option would be to do twenty minutes three times per week. A last option is to take a half day, once per week, if a daily regimen is too difficult. Of course, you may have to be flexible because life changes every day. But we must start putting ourselves as top, A+, number one priority because our body needs it!

Unfortunately, it is only at our most difficult times in life that we look outward, at a higher being, for help. We might have conversations with God in our minds without even realizing it. We don't have to wait till then. It might just be time for us to get ahead of our reckless way of life and take a realistic view of ourselves, what is important in life, our beliefs, our actions, and our mental and spiritual health and how it impacts our bodies. Taking the time to reconnect with the spirit you have been given, your God, being grateful for who you are, and thinking positively about what gifts you have, are key factors to concentrate on during your personal time. Taking this time away from the daily stressors and details of life, greatly reduces stress. If you have difficulty guiding your own thoughts, there are many great CDs and online videos that can be used for relaxation, prayer and positive thought.

There is substantial scientific evidence that sustained stress can have a negative impact on overall health. Stress can affect your emotions, behaviors and even some physiologic responses.[256] Not only does stress increase cortisol, it also increases adrenaline which uses up methyl groups that are normally utilized to break down estrogen. Stress is a proestro. This is you … making estrogen. Time to stop! (I know, Mrs. High Cortisol herself!)

Change 3: AHHH SLEEP

This *is* the S.L.E.E.P. Method after all. You didn't think we could get through this book without talking about sleep did you? One thing is for sure…we are all so tired all the time. Work is hard, life is hard and there are always a million things to do. It doesn't help to have little monkey climbing into bed in the mornings or middle of the night, but we all have active lives and responsibilities we have to make a conscious effort to work with. That is why it is crucial that we go to sleep at a decent time. We need to make sure we are getting the amount of sleep we need plus some time for interruptions. Sometimes it seems like this is the most difficult thing to do, even though it is one of the most important aspects of life. We can't think or act if we don't have enough sleep. Everyone is different, but most people know how much sleep they need. I need seven and a half hours but I know people who are fine with six hours. I try to allow for eight hours of sleep so I have time for bathroom breaks and child interruptions, as I know I can count on them to happen.

A good way to start getting more sleep if you are having difficulty, is to go to bed fifteen minutes earlier each night. A method that I like to use is reverse setting the alarm. You can set an alarm for a half hour prior to your bedtime. That will be your cue to start getting ready for bed.

One of the largest deterrents of sleep is television. Deprivation of television time is not necessarily a tortuous event for our bodies, although, with some people, you would think it might be. TV is mostly for the purpose of entertainment. My husband claims it is his meditation time because it takes his mind off daily stress. So, for all who claim TV is calming, that's fine. The main idea is; you want to stop watching television or using any computer screens at least two hours prior to bedtime. The lights activate signals in the brain through the eyes and don't allow melatonin, the sleep hormone, to kick in. Once I started getting to bed by 10pm, my body started getting sleepy at 8:30pm when I put my child to bed. It is possible to get used to an earlier bedtime. I used to be a night owl too.

Sleep is vitally important to decrease stress. As mentioned previously, stress can increase estrogens.

Change 4: EXERCISE

Exercise is another one of the most important things you can do to change your health. It reduces stress, builds muscle, strengthens the circulatory system, helps drain the lymphatic system of chemicals, keeps weight down and controls insulin levels. Exercising two to three times per week is enough to do all this.

As we age, being overweight increases estrogen and affects insulin levels, making it a good environment for breast cancer. Non-diabetic women with high insulin levels have twice the risk of breast cancer recurrence and three times the risk of death as women with low insulin levels. It has been proven in many scientific studies that women who have a higher body mass index (BMI), have a significantly increased risk of developing breast cancer. One of the reasons why is because fat cells actually produce estrogen.[257] Having a high amount of fat cells increases estrogen and/or insulin, makes it difficult to slow growth of abnormal cells. Since exercise directly coincides with weight, we can make it our goal to exercise in order to keep fat cells at a nominal level.

Conversely, it is agreed upon that exercise can decrease breast cancer risk. [258] Scientific studies are now linking this directly to changes in estrogen metabolism. Exercise increases protective 2OHE1 and decreases the proestro, 16a-OHE1.[257] Women who have breast cancer

[257] Smith AJ et al. May 2013 *Cancer Epidemiol Biomarkers* Prev "The effects of aerobic exercise on estrogen metabolism in healthy premenopausal women".
[258] Bernstein L et al. 1994 *Journal of the National Cancer Institute* "Physical exercise activity and reduced risk of breast cancer in young women".

and exercise one to five hours a week have shown a reduced recurrence risk by 6 to 58%. Exercise is also known to decrease inflammation (another side effect of weight gain) which as you heard before has shown to promote breast cancer, especially the HER2 type.

In 2013, I decided to try Phil Campbell's PEAK fitness program. What's great about this program is that it only takes 20 minutes, 3X per week. The first part involves interval training on a tread mill or elliptical machine or whatever machine works for you two times per week. The second part, weight lifting, is done one time per week and doesn't have you doing a million reps, which if you're like me, is totally boring. I can get through weight lifting in 15 minutes. Not too bad, huh? This type of program gives you the minimum exercise needed to keep your insulin levels down, lymphatics draining and body in shape. It is not necessarily for those who are trying to lose weight or gain muscle.

Craig Ballantyne has a training program that works well for gaining muscle. I tried this in 2014 just to change things up. It is called "Turbulence Training". You don't need any workout machines or gym memberships for this. You may need some hand weights and an exercise ball. It does require a lot of repetitions however. Even if you only do two reps, that is better than zero!

Lastly, there are workout videos and even online group training. This year I tried the 21Day Fix by *Beach Body* and am having great results, especially feeling stronger and healthier. There is no excuse these days for not having some sort of exercise routine!

Change 5: LYMPHATIC MASSAGE AND DRAINAGE

Recently, eye catching articles have been popping up in Facebook about how you can reduce breast cancer by having your breasts massaged. Believe it or not, there may be some truth to this. Lymphatic massage and slight pressure helps guide estrogens and chemicals out of the breast area, as well as makes changes to the cellular make-up of cancer cells. Choosing the right bra can also affect the lymphatics and is important to make good decisions in this regard.

In order to understand how the lymphatics can help deter breast cancer, we must understand their function. *The Mayo Clinic Breast Cancer Book*, written in 2012, describes the composition of breasts this way:[259]

"Blood vessels and lymph vessels run throughout your breasts. Blood nourishes breast cells. Lymph vessels carry a clear fluid called lymph, which contains immune system cells and drains waste products from tissues. (Who knew we had "waste" in our breasts?) *Lymph vessels lead to pea-sized collections of tissue called lymph nodes. Most of the lymph vessels in the breast lead to lymph nodes under the arm."*

Preventative steps such as exercise, avoiding use of patentable hormones and doing an estrogen detox supplement routine will all cause your breasts to slough off estrogens out of fat cells. You can help push these out by helping the lymph flow. An article by Jon Barron of the *Baseline of Health Foundation* says that lymphatic massage can increase the volume of lymph flow by as much as twenty times![260] It helps move the lymphatics and that makes the breast tissue healthier and less toxic. This can be important because guiding any estrogenic substances out can speed up the elimination process.

Not only does lymphatic massage increase lymph flow, a gentle pressure applied to the breast can help prevent breast cancer in a couple other ways. Pressure may also help return abnormal cells to a normal state. Scientists at the University of California, Berkeley found in 2012 that mechanical forces to cells can actually revert and stop growth of cancer cells.[261] They did not necessary recommend that we all need

[259] *The Mayo Clinic Breast Cancer Book*, 2012 Lynn C. Hartmann, M.D. and Charles L Loprinzi, M.D. p 45.

[260] Jon Barron of *Baseline of Health Foundation* July 2006 www.jonbarron.org/article/optimizing-your-lymph-system

[261] *UC Berkeley News Center* Dec 2012 University of California, Berkeley and the

to start wearing compression bras as a treatment, but it does show that gentle pressure to the breast will not hurt the cancer cells and it may even help! Lastly, applying pressure will help you become aware of any lumps. Both thermography and self-exam are vital ways for you to determine if your lumps are shrinking or growing!

You can look at the next diagram to see where the lymphatic vessels are located. It is easiest to do lymphatic massage in the shower or bath with soapy water, daily, while undergoing the S.L.E.E.P. Method. You can gently push from the nipple up and out to the side. For larger breasts you may need to push from the nipple down to the bottom as well. Be careful not to press too hard because that can cause abnormal cell growth.

Lawrence Berkeley National Laboratory study found compression of breast cancer cells can cause them to return to a normal state.

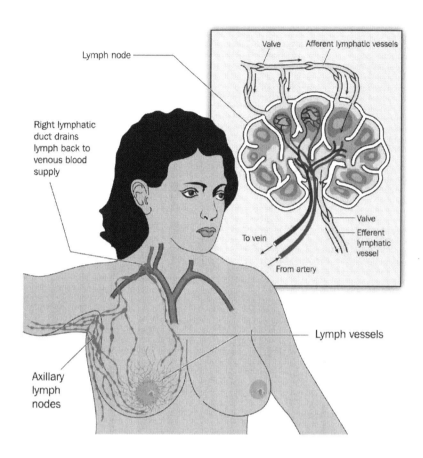

If you have been diagnosed with fibrocystic breasts, this step may be painful. If so, skip this step. Fibrocystic breast disease is not really a disease at all, but actually is pain due to swelling, firmness, or lumpy breasts. Since we are working on getting rid of lumps, most women have improvement in their pain from doing these steps, especially with iodine use.

Bra, Bra, Bra

Under-wire bras can interfere with lymphatic drainage. Scientific evidence does not support the abandonment of wire bras, but it goes without saying that wired bras are uncomfortable anyway. It may not be that difficult to give them up. After breast surgery, doctors recommend wireless bras for comfort and to increase healing. The same recommendation can be applied here. At least most days, you can wear a comfortable bra knowing that it may be helping your lymphatics drain.

I still wear the wired and padded bras when I want to look better in clothing. It really is just whether you have a societal obligation that you feel you need to adhere to or not. As for me, it's more about personal confidence. I feel better about myself when my chest looks peppier, as do most women, but I certainly don't feel bad about myself just because I look flat chested or not as shapely with a sports bra.

I searched everywhere for the right bra. I ended up finding a 100% cotton wireless bras made by Jockey. I also found some cotton tank style bras at The Gap and Walmart. It seems it is in style now to wear sports bras everywhere. This fad has come at the right time!

I couldn't find many bras without polyester or latex. These synthetic substances make me itch. As long as your skin does not have a reaction to polyester or latex, there are many choices out there for you to go wireless! It is important to make sure you are not irritating your skin as this may cause inflammation and will certainly not be a healing experience for your breasts.

Chapter 14

E is for EAT GOOD FOOD

Battle Step E is when we stop feeding proestros to our body and replace them with good healthy body food. Proestro-laced foods have animal hormones, chemicals and substances like pesticides that increase estrogen. This step may be the most challenging, but it is one of the most important changes you can make to reduce your body's burden of proestros. Once you get into a routine of purchasing good foods, there is nothing about it that increases your time quotient. The only difference may be a slight increase in grocery budget.

When scientists link certain foods to breast cancer and the results are publicized, we start to see food intake trends change. If we look at the science a little closer and then eliminate all the foods that are linked with breast cancer, we are left with organic fruit and vegetables. It is easy to come to conclusions based on single studies and then look at one aspect or a physical thing, such as a piece of meat, and say "this is what causes cancer". But the reality is, it's what is *in* the food, the way it's processed and our eating patterns that contribute to the cause of cancer. If we stick to eating a variety of good foods without chemicals, hormones, pesticides, or over processing, there would be nowhere near the amount of cancer there is today. Going back to earlier times in our history, we used lard to cook and we ate bread, meat and vegetables, and breast cancer was not nearly as prevalent.

Changing and understanding our diet requires us to reflect on the way we have been eating in the past. I spent many of my early years eating Hot Pockets® and ramen noodle soup. This kind of long term diet is just not healthy. Eventually, disease shows up and we realize it might be a good idea to change the way we eat. If you have eaten large amounts of carbohydrates in the past, it may be a good idea to go without them or decrease them for a while. If you have eaten lots of red meat, it may be a good idea to significantly decrease or remove your red meat intake for a while. It's all about balance. We can look at daily balance, but we can also look at balance in terms of our total lifetime.

Fat is a large portion of our diet and is in most foods we eat. When it comes to fats, there is some controversy over which fats are good and which are bad. Bad fats have been linked to clogging of the arteries, weight gain and of course, breast cancer. How fats function in an animal or in humans can vary based on how the fat was made. So even though some fats may be considered bad, they may not be in certain instances. Again, we will see that it is not necessarily the fat that is bad, but what is *in* the fat that is not good for us.

In this section, I have condensed the information to make diet change easier. There are six categories of our diet to focus on for breast cancer prevention. For the busy woman who doesn't have much time to cook, much less scour all the grocery shelves for weird ingredients, I have included in Chapter 17 a food product list, grocery store food lists, and some sample healthy foods that are easy to make or are pre-packaged.

I am still amazed at how changing my diet changes the way I feel. My energy increases significantly when eating the right foods. Not only that, but my body has actually trained my mind into recognizing the physical feelings associated with food that is bad for me. Now, I can't stomach the idea of eating desserts laden with sugar. I can't eat more than two pieces of pizza without feeling disgusted. My brain now tells me what it doesn't want. It is kind of like learning to play guitar. At first it is tedious and difficult. Then it becomes easier and eventually you don't have to consciously think about it. Fingers do the playing; mind stays out of it. Body does the digesting and tells us when to say no.

There are many literary resources that may be helpful to breast cancer prevention using a more healthful diet. Food Babe is an online resource and advocate for getting chemicals out of our food in the US. She has led the way by going directly to large food corporations and getting people to sign petitions against the additives in foods made by those corporations. She has good information about food using online sources and blogs, if you prefer surfing the internet.

A book called *The Whole-Food Guide for Breast Cancer Survivors: A Nutritional Approach to Preventing Recurrence* by Edward Bauman Med Ph.D., Helayne Waldman MS EdD and Donald I Abrams M.D., is a good source for understanding diet and how it relates to breast cancer. Also, *The Breast Cancer Prevention Diet* by Dr. Bob Arnot is easily available in used book stores or libraries. Even one of the oldest books around recommends healthy eating. I found it interesting that even *The Bible* states in Isaiah 55 "Why spend your money on food that does not give you strength?" Maybe we just need to listen to His advice.

EAT 1: ORGANIC FRUIT and VEGETABLES; Avoid Pesticides and GMOs

Pesticides

Pesticides can mimic the action of estrogen in the body. As you have seen already, there are many studies that link pesticides, such as atrazine, as an endocrine disrupter. It goes without saying that we would want to eliminate as much pesticide laced foods from our diet as possible. Pesticides can be found in our food and water. We can eliminate these from our diet and water sources by becoming aware of their existence and then utilizing a few tools.

One way to do this is to eat organic food or buy meat, fish, peanuts, fruit and vegetables directly from pesticide free farms. Eating all organic may prove to be difficult at times since not all grocers carry organic, pesticide free produce and farms may not be nearby and it is more expensive. For this reason, it would help to thoroughly rinse any non-organic foods prior to eating.

Removing pesticides from our drinking water can be done by using certain filters. I included a comparison on filters for you later in the

Eradicate section of the S.L.E.E.P. Method. Using supplements, as discussed in this book, such as MSM, milk thistle and probiotics, can help your body be more effective at processing out pesticides.

The Environmental Working Group tested 48 fruit and vegetable categories for pesticide content. The following twelve had the highest pesticide load and would be the ones you would focus on buying organic. For vegetables that you eat regularly, you may also want to buy organic. For instance, if you eat broccoli frequently during the week, you may want to get organic broccoli.

Apples
Celery
Cherry
Cucumber
Grapes
Hot Peppers
Nectarines (imported)
Peaches
Potato
Spinach
Strawberries
Sweet bell peppers
Kale
Collard Greens
Summer Squash

On the other hand, the following tested low, so you will probably be okay to purchase these not organic. However, keep in mind certain ones will be GMO; for example, corn and papaya

Asparagus
Avocado
Bananas
Cabbage
Cantaloupe

Sweet corn (non-GMO)
Eggplant
Grapefruit
Kiwi
Mango
Mushrooms
Onions
Papayas (most Hawaiian is GMO)
Pineapple
Sweet peas (frozen)
Sweet potatoes

Genetically Modified Organisms

GMOs (also called transgenic), are a hot button issue these days. GMO foods are crops that have their genes changed to create breeds or strains of plants and animals that do not naturally occur. GMO crops are made this way to be less prone to pest infestation so that pesticide use may be reduced. Even though the use of GMO plants may reduce the need for pesticide use, many countries like Germany, United Kingdom, Spain, Italy, Greece, France, Sri Lanka, Thailand, China and Japan have put restrictions on GMO foods. To date, three US States have also approved bills to require labeling of GMO foods.

In order to understand the reasons why these countries are restricting GMO use, we need to understand how GMOs are created. Monsanto Company is the leading producer of genetically engineered seed and the herbicide glyphosate, which it markets under the "Roundup" brand. The seeds they genetically modify are pest resistant because they have "Roundup" integrated inside them. From what I understand, scientists have changed the genetic makeup for the pesticide so it cannot harm humans. For the farmer, this provides a crop that is disease and pest resistant, which increases production and therefore income. Of course you are not going to hear that some pesticide version is *in* the plant instead of *on* the plant. Countries have banned GMO use due to the many questions that remain regarding long term pesticide use inside of a plant.

Monsanto Company has patents on their GMO seeds. This, in itself, is becoming a threat to biodiversity because the seeds to these plants cannot reproduce. Could these plants be a contributor to cancer or reproduction problems in society? According to most studies on www.pubmed.org, this is not the case. However, there are several things that are left out or noticeably missing from the online studies.

A few GMO rat tests were multi-generational but they did not list how long each generation was tested. A few studies I reviewed were on rats using GMO rice or soy and were ninety days long. These rats were only fed 30 to 60% GMO foods. Many questions still remain. Why didn't they feed the rats 80% GMO foods? Why haven't GMO foods been tested longer than ninety days? Why haven't they tested this food on humans? After all, we are already eating it.

As Dr. Joseph Mercola points out in his article on GMOs, nineteen studies showed signs of organ disruption. Accessing the actual studies may prove difficult. The studies on www.pubmed.gov are mostly reviews and conclusion of studies, not the actual, full documentation of studies. Recently, scientists wanted to produce a paper on GMO studies, but had to get a court order and fill out official paperwork to even get a copy of research from Monsanto. It does not appear the scientists from Monsanto are making the research freely available for the casual layman or public to read. What kind of scientific research is it then? What are they hiding from us? Monsanto studies are nowhere to be found!

Of the GMO studies that I did find, only two were over ninety days long. One of these studies was performed in 2012 in Russia.[262] Surprisingly, after ninety days, the rats died, began to get sick or got tumors. This

---

[262] Seralini, GE et al Nov 2012 *Food Chem Toxicol* "Long term toxicity of a Roundup herbicide and a Roundup-tolerant genetically modified maize".

study was published in *Food and Chemical Toxicology*. Monsanto and scientists discounted the study citing that rats that typically develop cancer were used. Well, what happened to the control group then? That group did not develop cancer. I looked up the type of rats used in the study. *Sprague Dawley* rats turn out to be common rats used in many studies and the same rat used in the Monsanto studies! They are typical lab rats...nothing unusual there.

If you want to trust a food that is altered by a company that also manufacturers Roundup® and previously manufactured warfare herbicide Agent Orange, then most of the studies thus far would support it. I would rather bet on regular organic food and stay clear of anything related to hidden, questionable science or pesticides.

ResponsibleTechnology.org has created a *Non-GMO Shopping Guide* for free at www.NonGMOShoppingGuide.com in order to help you decipher what to buy. You can download it into a pdf or you can even get an app if you have an iPhone!

Organic Food

There are four categories of organic foods allowed by the USDA. They are:

100% Organic,
Organic
"Made with" Organic
Specific organic ingredients

We want to aim at buying 100% organic if possible. In "organic" labeled foods, there are non-organic ingredients allowed. These ingredients would have to be on the "National List of Allowed and Prohibited Substances" in organic livestock and crops. For example, a vaccine used for pink eye is allowed on the animals, arsenic is not allowed. These ingredients can only add up to a combined total of five percent of the non-organic content. Well, it's not perfect, but we can only do our best!

Not all stores offer 100% organic for everything. If you shop at a local farmer's market or butcher shop, you can find out directly from the vendor about pesticides, GMOs and hormones. Many farms are now offering "naturally grown", which may have better standards than organic does. Evidently every batch of food produced, is tested for pesticides. Just because something is labeled organic doesn't mean it has been tested for pesticides.

Fruit and Vegetables

One way to get organic is to grow your own organic vegetables in a garden. This is *not* the easy way, but it does save some money and makes finding a tomato easy during the growing season. It also counts toward your exercise routine! I am looking into making a hydroponic garden on my deck which involves no movement of heavy dirt! Now, I just have to glue some pipes together and drill some holes and I will be all set.

Another way to get organic vegetables is from a local farmer's market. Many times, local farms are not officially organic but they do claim that they do not use pesticides. Personally, I don't have time to make a zillion grocery store and farmer's market stops, so I buy organic from grocery stores. Wegmans, Trader Joes, Whole Foods, Harris Teeter and even Walmart are offering a wide array of organic produce.

EAT 2: LEAN GRASS FED MEAT; Avoid: Pesticides, Dioxins, Hormones, Omega-6, Saturated Fat and Artificial Trans-fats

Humans are omnivores. We are not meant to just eat vegetables like herbivores. We need to eat animal protein to survive because our bodies need amino acids. Herbivores have four stomachs to break down food because raw vegetables are very difficult to digest. For our single stomach, we need a combination of foods to help break them down.

There are several reasons typical meat, especially red meat, is associated with increased breast cancer risk. One, is that animals are fed pesticide laced grain. Two, is the hormones given to cattle and pork, is stored inside the fat and this fat is bad. Three, is that there are unbalanced quantities of fats typically found in meat. Fourth, is the high amount of iron in red meat.

Pesticides in Animals

Animals can have pesticides accumulate in their bodies from what they ingest. Cows, chickens and pigs may eat corn and hay with pesticides, which stay in their bodies. Because of this, we want to aim for eating animals that have been raised and finished, eating pesticide and GMO free grass, corn and hay. If a cow is eating untreated grass, you're not ingesting any GMOs or pesticides, which are proestros. I have personally worked for a cattle ranch and I know first-hand that there are still many farms that raise cattle on real land and not in "feed lots". These farmers do not inject their cattle with hormones, nor do they feed them corn or junk. They are fed hay and grass. For this reason, the meat you buy does not have to be certified organic, which can be quite expensive. You can still buy a cow directly from a farm or local butcher shop that carries grass fed beef to avoid pesticides in your meat.

Dioxins

There are seventy-five dibenzo-p-dioxins (PCDDs), seven of which are toxic. These dioxins are not actual pesticides themselves but are by-products of manufacturing pesticides, such as organochlorine. Agent Orange, the herbicide used in warfare to kill crops, contained dioxin. Pesticides like organochlorine are part of a larger chlorine industry which also manufactures bleaching paper, plastics and solvents and contribute to PCDDs. The largest issue with PCDDs is that they are not easily broken down in the environment.

Human ingestion of PCDDs is from meat, fish and dairy products, as PCDDs are picked up from soil, are not water soluble and are stored in animal fat. After you ingest these animals or animal products, PCDDs build up in your body fat, and are not easily excreted. The half-life is said to be seven to eight years and concentrations may increase five to tenfold from age 20 to age 60.

Finding out how long these PCDDs exist in our bodies was disheartening enough, and then I also found out that dioxins are in tampons. Tampons are made of cotton and cotton is sprayed with these pesticides. The FDA has stated that it only exists in small amounts in tampons and is not harmful. However, knowing that the skin inside the vaginal wall is thin, any small amounts of dioxins may most certainly be absorbed into the blood stream over the course of a woman's life. It would be a good idea to purchase organic cotton tampons and pads to avoid this and other chemicals in tampons.

What PCDDs do to the body has been demonstrated through many animal studies. PCDDs promote cancer growth, but do not necessarily promote estrogen. In humans, PCDD has proven to affect sexual development and, in cases of high exposure due to work environment, cause cancer. The EPA has categorized dioxin as a "likely human carcinogen"

Dioxins such as PCDD will **not** be listed on any food product ingredients, so we have to be aware of their existence when sourcing our meat, fish and dairy.

Hormones

Believe it or not, 80% of cows are raised in Concentrated Animal Feeding Operations (CAFOs) their entire life and are not given their natural environment or diet. They are fed grains instead of grass which increases the acid in their stomachs. An acidic environment is what e-coli need to survive. Due to this, and the way these animals are raised, they also have a higher risk of pathogenic contamination. Because of risk of contamination, farmers have to use low dose antibiotics to keep these pathogens at bay. These factors all add up to mean typical red meats are high in chemical trans-fats and bovine hormones, which may increase your risk of breast cancer. [263] [270] Bovine hormones are stored in the animal's fat, which is most likely the reason there is this breast cancer association.

Even animals raised on pasture may eventually be sold to the slaughter house, as the farmer may not slaughter onsite. You may want to get it before it goes there, because that's when they are fattened up in a "feed lot", three months prior to slaughter. Beef finished on corn and grain are known to have unhealthy fats that are linked with all sorts of health problems, so finishing them with grain may have a similar effect. Similar to a CAFO, in a feed lot, there are more bacteria, so animals are given antibiotics. Again, they may also be given hormones to fatten them up.

Omega-6

We know our body needs fat to survive and we get most our fats from meat, oils, nuts, and dairy. When thinking in terms of fats, it is a good idea to consume them in the same ratio that our own tissues contain. Our fat tissue is mostly made of saturated and monounsaturated fat. Since most animal fat contains both saturated and monounsaturated fat, we can easily attain these fats as long as we are not eating a

---

[263] Thordarson G et al. Oct 2004 Breast Cancer Res Treat "Mammary tumorigenesis in growth hormone deficient spontaneous dwarf rats; effects of hormonal treatments".

vegetarian diet. Polyunsaturated fats (PUFAs) are a very small part of our fat tissue and we do not need to eat that much. PUFAs include omega-6 and omega-3. Intake of monounsaturated fats and omega-3 fats are associated with decreased risk of breast cancer.[264]

The problem is, our society as a whole is eating way too much PUFAs. Vegetable oils are high in PUFA, especially omega-6. Ingestion of excessive vegetable oil, nuts, eggs and fatty meats will be enough to throw the body off balance and cause many long-term problems. It is crucial to have PUFAs in balance. When consumed in excess, PUFAs can cause chronic inflammation, which suppresses the immune system. Since PUFA is another very important source of inflammation in the body, we need to keep it balanced to prevent breast cancer. We do need small amounts of PUFA to modulate and regulate inflammatory eicosanoids. If you are eating a healthy balanced diet, you will not have a deficiency in PUFAs.

PUFAs should not be eaten at the same time as fruit or anything with fructose in it. They can create toxic by-products which can then cause all sorts of damage. This means that if we are drinking a protein shake with almond milk, we may want to avoid having any fruit in it. Almonds have a high amount of omega-6. When eaten in high quantities, PUFAs also create high cholesterol, which is not a good situation for the heart.

One of the PUFAs, omega-3, only needs to be eaten in small quantities. High levels can also cause problems. Lately, there is concern about getting the proper ratio of omega-3 to omega-6 from food sources, so people are overdoing omega-3. The key is to lower omega-6, and slightly raise up omega-3. The proper ratio of omega-6 to omega-3 is around 1:1 or 1:2. Ingesting omega-3 from raw seeds, fish or fish oil is the best way to raise omega-3.

---

[264] Khodoarahmi M and Azadbakht L Jan 2014 *Int J Prev Med* "The Association Between Different Kinds of Fat Intake and Breast Cancer Risk in Women".

Saturated and Trans Fats

The FDA requires that saturated fats and trans fats be listed on food labels. This is due to a history of saturated fats and trans fats being linked to higher LDL cholesterol levels that increase the risk of coronary heart disease. A review of fat intake in Jan of 2014 said that scientific evidence shows a link between saturated fats and increased breast cancer risk. The USDA recommends limiting saturated fat to 20g per day. Other experts don't focus on the amount of saturated fat, but from where it is sourced. They say that eating saturated fats from healthy grass fed animals is actually good for us!

There is no argument that there is a reduced risk of breast cancer associated with omega-3 polyunsaturated fats (PUFA). [265] It would be ideal to lower fats that are high in omega 6, chemical trans-fats and saturated fats from regular processed meats. This means we can still eat red meats, as long as they are grass fed.

Here is a table so you can see the relevant fat values of meats. Grass fed beef and venison look pretty good in terms of fats compared to everything else!

It is important to know there is a difference between chemical trans-fats and natural trans fats. Natural trans fats are produced in the stomach of some animals. These trans-fats may be found in small amounts in dairy and meat products and are not known to be harmful. Artificial trans fats (or trans fatty acids) are created by an industrial process that adds hydrogen to liquid vegetable oils to make them more solid.

---

[265] Khodarahmi M and Azadbakht L Jan 2014 *Int J Prev Med* "The Association Between Different Kinds of Fat Intake and Breast Cancer Risk in Women".

FAT CONTENT IN MEAT

Meat 3 to 4oz	Omega 6	Omega 3	Saturated Fat
Grass fed beef (lean)	90mg	23mg	2-5g
Lamb	150-3000mg	100-1200mg	3.5-7g
Venison	220mg	100mg	1g
Bison (grass fed)	200-300mg	80mg	3.49g
Beef grain fed (lean)	300mg	10-30mg	2-8g
Pork (lean)	300mg	10mg	1-2g
Duck breast wild	510mg	10mg	1g
Turkey light meat	550g	20-60mg	.43g
Chicken light meat	690mg	76mg	1g
Veal	1000-2500mg	140mg	2.37g
Chicken thigh meat	1890mg	120-150mg	2.36g
Turkey meat and skin	2940mg	280mg	7.5
Chicken dark meat and skin	3040mg	190-240mg	4.47g
Pork Belly	5020mg	480mg	3-5.48g

These hydrogenated oils are used for salad dressings, mayonnaise and fried foods and contain chemical trans fats. It is critical to avoid all of these types of foods. Even though trans fats may not be listed on the label, processed foods still may contain them up to .5g per serving. The

USDA recommends limiting trans fats to 2g per day and many other authorities recommend eliminating it altogether.

According to Chris Kresser, an integrative medicine practitioner, the trans fats in grass fed meat and dairy have different chemical structures and effects on the body than chemical trans fats from oils. These natural trans fats, known as CLA, are three to five times higher in grass fed meats and have been shown to lower cancer risk in scientific experiments and case control studies. CLA works by blocking the growth and spread of tumors. Chris cites five studies to prove it. We should not have to be concerned with eating meat with natural trans fats. [266]

The worst component we find in the fat of our meats are hormones, pesticides and chemical trans fats. Therefore, the most important thing to consider when buying meat is that it is lean and hormone and pesticide free. We can do this by purchasing organic or grass fed meat.

When you do eat red meat, marinating before cooking and not cooking it on the grill is recommended. Cooking meat on the grill at high temperatures has proven to create carcinogens that contribute to cancer development.

Iron

In addition to pesticide and GMO fed meat, as well as hormone and fat concerns, there is concern that red meat is high in iron. If iron levels are too high in the body, it can lead to cancer by triggering free radicals and inflammation, which in turn, can stimulate cancer growth. If you eat vegetables with your red meat, that decreases absorption of iron. This is just one of the few examples proving that we are meant to eat an assortment of foods, not just meat, and not just vegetables! Limiting red meat to grass fed or organic is a good way to keep fat stored

---

[266] www.chriskesser.com/can-som-trans-fats-be-healthy

hormones out of your body. You do not need to have red meat guilt! As long as the meat is grass fed, you can eat normal amounts of red meat.

Acquisition of Grass Fed Meat

I recently ordered 1/8 of a grass fed cow from a local farm. I found a place that let me order what they call a "beef box". The cost was less than buying regular meat at the grocery store and I didn't have to buy ½, ¼ or even a whole cow! The place I ordered from only uses fly spray near the cow's eyes during fly season for humane reasons...no other pesticides or GMO anything. Well at least it is a heck of lot less pesticides than what I am typically ingesting! I am set for at least two or three months and will spend less time shopping, which is a big plus in my book!

Chickens are not typically treated with hormones, as most packaging states, but we may want to think about how the chicken meat is preserved and what the chickens are eating. Most chickens eat GMO feed. Unless you are buying organic or chickens fed *Non-GMO Certified* feed, you may be ingesting some pesticides along with your chicken. Here is a website where you check to see if retailers or products are non-GMO certified: www.nongmoproject.org.

If you are having difficulty finding hormone, pesticide and GMO free beef, chicken, lamb or pork in your area, here is a website where you can find some local farms: www.eatwild.com. Another option is to order your meat online. www.grasslandbeef.com is an example of a group of farms working together to get beef and lamb delivered to you.

If ordering meat online, or going to your local farmer is not an option for you, you can find organic meats at Trader Joes and Whole Foods. I cheat sometimes and get chicken that is not organic but is labeled "natural". "Natural" means that the product is minimally processed. It still may have preservatives and the animal may eat GMO products, so it is only slightly better than regular meats.

When buying chicken, it is important to realize that free range just means that the animal has access to the outdoors. It has nothing to do with what is in the food. So, if you care about how the animal is treated, this one is for you, but it does nothing for *your* body.

Lucky for us, my husband enjoys hunting and brings home venison and wild turkey for three seasons of the year. Now this is a good way to get low fat, grass fed meat! Of course, if the deer is from a suburban or farming area, there is no way to know for sure that it is eating pesticide free vegetation, but I would bet that most deer are eating better than cows eating grain in "feed lots".

EAT 3: WILD CAUGHT FISH with OMEGA-3; **Avoid PCBs and Omega 6**

Fish on the other hand, live downstream from farm water runoff and get pesticides and PCBs dumped on them from many different sources. You may have heard of fish dying from contaminated waters. This is from PCB and pesticide run off.

It is difficult to prove or know what you are getting when you buy fish. Acquiring fish from clean waters is what we want to aim for, if possible, but may be difficult to locate. Fish found in rivers upstream would most likely have less pollution in them. Any body of water where there is not a large people population, like the Amazon, would also be less polluted. The Northern Canada lakes and the Arctic, and Antarctic waters are among the cleanest in the world. Oceans tend to be a large dumping ground for air pollution and land run-off. Also, ocean water moves around quite a bit due to water currents, so pollution can be found throughout the oceans of the world.

Speaking of fresh water animals, when we bought my son a hermit crab, it came with a little instruction booklet. It specifically stated that hermit crabs should only be fed organic fruit or treats. One can only reason that a small organism cannot process or handle pesticides like our bodies can, without dying quickly. We humans just take a bit longer.

Omega-3 Fish

If you are like most people, you do eat *some* fish, which will contribute to your intake of omega-3, even if it is just flounder. However, most fish these days are farmed at sea in small pens or tanks, which is not the healthiest condition. These fish end up with an unhealthy balance of omega-6 to omega-3 ratio. Raising these fish in farms allows the farmer to get around timing and quantity regulations that are in place for wild caught fish. Even fresh water fish like cat fish and trout are being farmed. Still, wild fish are affected by pesticide and PCB run-off from farms. Unfortunately, our healthy fish supply is dwindling.

The safest sources of omega-3 rich fish are small to medium-size cold water fish like anchovies, sardines, trout, wild salmon and mussels. Some of these may be acquired tastes and may not be on your list of favorite choices of seafood. I know they aren't mine! I don't eat them, except for the occasional salmon or trout. Seafood to avoid are swordfish, king mackerel, and tilefish, which are large and live long lives. Longer living fish have time to store up more PCBs, dioxins and mercury. The more common white flaky fish like tilapia and flounder do not have as much omega-3, but they do have some and they are generally safer to eat, as long as they are wild caught.

Polychlorinated Biphenyls (PCBs)

Even though PCBs (polychlorinated biphenyls) were banned from being manufactured in 1979, they are still in our environment today. One of the places you can still find PCBs are on huge electric transformers, voltage regulators and bushings at substations. In the home, you may find them in fluorescent light ballasts, cable insulation, ceiling and wall insulation, paint, caulking and floor finishes.

Consumer products containing PCBs are disposed of and then make it to landfills or poorly maintained hazardous waste treatment facilities. Rain then washes PCBs into the ground and this is where they stay because they do not easily break down. PCBs may continue to cycle between air, water and soil for a long time and travel long distances. This makes it very difficult to get rid of PCBs.

Almost all fish contain PCBs. Where PCBS have accumulated, they are found in higher amounts in fish. The PCBs in fish and sediment also happen to be more toxic than PCBs that are released into the environment from factories. PCBs can also be found on the above ground portion of plants and food crops.

So, how serious a problem *are* PCBs? PCBs are considered probable human carcinogens by the EPA, The International Agency for Research on Cancer, The National Toxicology Program and the National Institute for Occupational Safety and Health. PCBs are one of the most widely studied environmental contaminants. Both animal studies and human population studies on PCB workers show that PCBs cause liver and skin cancer. Some PCBs are said the have dioxin like effects.[267]

PCBs don't make for a good hormone situation either for most the population. They have been found to be present in high levels in the breasts of breast cancer patients.[268] No direct correlation to breast cancer specifically has been made as of yet. It is associated with a host of other effects in the immune system, the reproductive system, the nervous system and the endocrine system in animals. Even at low doses, PCBs affect the immune system and are carcinogenic. The immune system is crucial in fighting any kind of cancer.

PCBs will **not** be listed on any food product ingredients, so we have to be aware of their existence when drinking water, eating fish and foods

---

[267] Brody JG et al. June 2007 *Cancer* "Environmental pollutants and breast cancer: epidemiologic studies".
[268] Ellsworth RE Apr 2015 *Environ Res* "Abundance and distribution of polychlorinated biphenyls (PCBs) in breast tissue."

or when remodeling our homes. PCBs can be filtered out of water, which I will discuss at the end of the Eradicate section.

Dioxins, toxaphene and dieldrin, as well as mercury can also be found in our fish. It is a good idea to limit your fish intake and verify the source. Wild caught will be better, but even wild fish are contaminated. If you are eating fish, it's a good idea to keep it to once or twice per week. You may take kelp or *Modifilan* with it to help separate and remove mercury out from the body.

Omega-6

When cooking fish, we will most likely use some sort of oil or butter. We do not want to counter the very omega-3 we are trying to ingest with omega-6. More recently developed saturated fats like margarine, soybean oil, sunflower oil, corn oil, canola oil and safflower oil use toxic solvents to extract the oil from the seeds. Their high omega-6 content can unbalance the ratio of omega-6s to omega-3s. Even Wikipedia says this:

"A high consumption of oxidized polyunsaturated fatty acids (PUFAs), which are found in most types of vegetable oil, may increase the likelihood that postmenopausal women will develop breast cancer."

Better oil choices are cold-pressed oils made without the use of chemicals or heat to extract the oil. They include olive oil, palm kernel oil and coconut oil. These oils are lower in omega-6, but they can still be high in saturated fat. If the oils are from organic sources, then the saturated fat content may not matter as much.

You can see from the following chart below which oils are better. Keep in mind this table is based on 3.5oz of oil which is approximately 7 tablespoons of oil. Hopefully, you will not be ingesting that amount each day! You can see why coconut oil is all the rave right now with lower grams of saturated fat and omega-6. High oleic sunflower oil may be another good option, but we need to watch for trans fats here.

A good fat can become bad if heat, light or oxygen damages it. Oils high in PUFAs, such as flaxseed oil, must be refrigerated and kept in an opaque container. If an oil smells or tastes rank or bitter, it should not be used. Cooking at high heat with some oils, such as olive oil, can damage the fat. Coconut oil, lard and clarified butter are not easily damaged and are okay to cook at high temperatures.

The American diet consists of a lot of fat. We have butter on toast or eat eggs and bacon in the morning. We use some vegetable oil dressing on a salad for lunch, along with some sort of meat or we mix some mayonnaise in a chicken or egg salad. Dinner we fry things up in the pan with oil or add oil to the meatloaf, meatballs or top a salad with some more oil. For snacks, we eat nuts or crackers with cheese or peanut butter. If you take a close look, it's fat at every meal and snack! We must be cognizant of the type of fats and amounts of we are eating or our health could get away from us.

Omega-3 supplements

Omega-3 supplements come in a variety of forms such as fish oil, krill oil and flaxseed oil. Fish oil is known to be more easily processed by the body than flaxseed. Like fish, fish oil supplements can also be contaminated. It is important to avoid products that do not list the source of their omega-3s. Look for the total amount of EPA and DHA on the label. Choose supplements that are mercury and PCB free and have been independently tested to be free of these and other toxins. You can choose the amount of omega-3 milligrams you take based on how many omega-6s you ingest.

FAT CONTENT IN OIL

Plant fats and oils 3.5oz (100g)	Omega-6	Omega-3	Saturated Fat
Clarified Butter or Ghee	2247mg	1447mg	61.9
Palm Kernel oil	1.6g	0	78.14g
Coconut oil	1.8g	0	12g
Butter	2.2g	1417mg	49.35g
Cocoa butter	2.8g	100mg	57.24g
Suet/Beef Mutton	3.1g	600mg	51.9g
Sunflower (high oleic)	3.6g	192mg	10.88g
Olive oil	9.8g	761mg	13.1g
Lard (pig and bacon)	10.2g	1000mg	35.38g
Avocado oil	12.5g	957mg	12.1g
Flaxseed oil	12.7g	53.3g	8.95g
Safflower oil (high oleic)	14.3g	0	5.95g
Peanut oil	31.7g	0	19.88g
Sesame oil	41.3g	300mg	14.1
Soybean oil	50.2g	7g	7.51g
Walnut oil	52.9g	10.4g	9.56g
Corn/Canola oil	53.5g	1g	7.46g
Sunflower oil (linoleic)	65.7g	0	6.51g

EAT 4: WHEY PROTEIN and GREEK YOGURT; Avoid Hormone and Lactose Dairy

Whey protein is awesome for our bodies. We actually start out drinking it. Breast milk contains 70% whey protein. Now, we don't have easy access to breast milk, nor do we want to drink breast milk as adults, so the best source is from by-products when making cheese and this typically comes in the form of a powder.

There are many benefits of whey protein: a quick meal when you are in a hurry, a great fortifier after a workout, a liver detoxifier, an immune system booster, and it even helps with anti-aging! Whey protein powder only contains 1g of saturated fat and total fat is low, so we don't have to worry about causing fat related health issues.

According to Dr. Joseph Mercola, glutathione (GSH) levels are always low in breast cancer patients. You can get natural GSH from animal foods, and whey protein. He suggests 5 to 40gms per day. A scientific study in Istanbul, Turkey showed that rats with colon cancer did not get as large tumors if they were fed whey protein.[269]

Finding a whey protein shake with all the "right stuff" can be challenging. There are several things to consider when shopping for whey protein. According to Dr. Joseph Mercola, we want a shake without isolates. Isolates do not dissolve or digest easily and can cause damage long term. Second, we want a protein derived from grass fed cow's milk to make sure we are drinking a product free from pesticides. Thirdly, we want a product that does not use harsh processes that remove alkaline minerals. Lastly, we want a product made without sugar, sugar substitutes or soy. It turns out, this may be asking for a lot!

---

[269] Attaallah W et al. Oct 2012 *Pathol Oncol* Res "Whey protein versus whey protein hydrolysate for the protection of azoxymethane and dextran sodium sulfate induced colonic tumors in rats".

I was drinking a whey protein shake, until I realized it had both whey protein concentrate, isolate and soy! I decided to go on a search for whey protein concentrate from grass fed cows sweetened with Stevia or no sweetener...and of course none of the bad stuff, heavy metals or soy. I found a few others besides Dr. Joseph Mercola's whey protein.

One is *Whey Natural* at www.wheynaturalusa.com. Second is *Vital Whey* which sells at www.amazon.com or www.wellwisdom.com. Third is *Naked Whey* which also sells on www.amazon.com and other places. The most inexpensive per serving was the 2.5-pound bag of Vital Whey on Amazon for approximately $1.30 per serving. Prices change so make sure you check before you buy!

Another type of protein shake I recently ran into was a beef protein shake. This sounds awful but I will probably give it a try as long as they are grass fed organic cows!

Hormone and Lactose Dairy

Milk products have hormones like rBGH (recombinant bovine growth hormone) and rBST (recombinant bovine somatropin), which have been linked to breast and other cancers.[263] These hormones are carried inside the fat cells of dairy products. Higher fat dairy products will carry more of these hormones. A study in 1996 showed that there was an increase in insulin growth factor-1 (IGF-1) in cow's milk when they are given rBGH. EGF-1 is further increased with pasteurization.[270] This incriminates regular milk as a risk factor for breast cancer and gastrointestinal cancers and gives us a good reason to avoid high fat milk, sour cream and cottage cheese. Organic dairy means the cow from where it was derived, did not eat pesticide laden food to pass on to you and was not given any hormone treatment. Organic dairy will be free of these hormones.

---

[270] Epstein SS 1996 *Int J health Ser* "Unlabeled milk from cows treated with biosynthetic growth hormones: a case of regulatory abdication".

Another reason to avoid dairy is because, for some people, the lactose is difficult to digest. According to various sources, up to 75% of people worldwide have the enzyme needed (lactase) to break down lactose. This means that at least 25% don't have enough lactase. You can resolve lactase bloating and gas by taking a lactase enzyme, typically in pill form, when you drink milk or eat cheese.

According to Dr. Natasha McBride, passing gas is a sign that digestion is not going well. If you notice you're a bit gassy or bloated after drinking milk, there is your sign that you don't have enough lactase! Even though we have not been taught this and we always laugh about it, gas is not good or "normal". Watch for gas after drinking milk or eating other dairy products. Dr. McBride also says milk is meant for babies and toddlers anyway. Even babies can have difficulty digesting milk and develop colic. Once you are an adult, your body does not process lactose as well.

Still, many of us would feel amiss if we could not have some milk in our life. Lactaid (lactose free) milk is not necessarily hormone free, so be careful thinking lactaid milk is the answer to all your milk problems. Organic Valley does make lactose free, organic milk. That's a mouthful, but there you can have your milk! You can go to www.organicvalley.coop/ to find out where this product is sold. This will ensure you are not getting extra hormones, pesticides or lactose that your body does not need.

Generally, milk is known for being rich in calcium, vitamin D and protein, all of which are good for your body and breast cancer prevention. It should also be noted that some dairy, like milk, has sugar in it. So be careful making milk your drink of choice. I was surprised to see five grams of sugar in ½ cup of milk, so make sure to count it towards your daily intake of sugar if you are calculating sugar.

There are substitutes for milk that may be quite healthy. I used to prefer unsweetened and flavorless almond milk. The taste is most similar to regular milk, it has more protein and calcium than regular milk and it doesn't cause gas. Then, I found out almonds are a type of goitrogen, which disrupts the production of thyroid hormones and interferes with iodine uptake of the thyroid. I have hypothyroid, so I am staying away from almond milk for now. Also, the more I drank it, the more I noticed it was difficult to digest. I started to get acid reflux when eating almonds in the same day. Coconut milk is what I use now in protein shakes and as a good substitute for regular milk in recipes. Unsweetened, flavorless also has a nice, pleasant taste! I try to keep it to 6oz or less of coconut milk. Coconuts have omega-6 in them!

Unlike some breast cancer prevention recommendations, I do not say avoid all dairy. Dairy is where we get most of our calcium (1000 mg recommended per day), vitamins D, A and K2. Studies show that dairy (except milk) may be associated with reduced risk of breast cancer. [271] Even if you are drinking almond milk, you will need some dairy. Perhaps the reason why many studies have shown that cheeses and dairy are protective against breast cancer is because vitamin D and calcium are protective.[272]

Fermented dairy, such as yogurt, is one of the great dairy products you can eat, especially if it is homemade and raw. Yogurt has plenty of good bacteria (probiotics) and the lactose is gone after fermentation because it is processed longer. Again, we will have to make sure it is from a hormone free cow. Organic, plain, unsweetened, Greek yogurt is a great alternative. It provides more protein than other yogurts. It is a nice snack before bedtime with some granola or banana and a tsp of honey.

Cheese is another dairy product to include in your diet. Because hard cheeses process for a longer time, the lactose is mostly eliminated. Cheeses with high vitamin content like Swiss, feta, mozzarella and

---

[271] Dong JY et al. May 2011 *Breast Cancer Res Treat* "Dairy consumption and risk of breast cancer: a meta-analysis of prospective cohort studies".

[272] Aro A et al. 2000 Nutr Cancer "Inverse association between dietary and serum conjugated linoleic acid and risk of breast cancer in postmenopausal women".

Gouda are excellent choices. Again, organic cheeses would be a better option and no fat or rBST free cheese would be a second option.

Recently, I found out that cheeses wrapped in plastic carry high levels of BPA. It seems like we are never going to win! If you can find cheeses wrapped in foil or wax paper, it would be much better. Organic eggs have ½ g less saturated fat per egg versus non organic eggs so there is another reason to eat organic!

EAT 5: FLAXEED and NUTS; **Avoid Unfermented Soy**

Nuts and Seeds

We probably don't associate nuts as a problem when it comes to breast cancer, but nuts have some of the highest counts of omega-6, even higher than most meats. A good alternative to eating nuts is to eat seeds. Two seeds that are high in omega-3 and low in omega-6 are flaxseed and chia seeds.

Flaxseed is also good if you are trying to increase healthy estrogens during menopause. It contains high amounts of omega-3, in addition to some weak estrogens which can take the place of stronger toxic estrogens. Flaxseed contains lignans, compounds in a plant that can be metabolized into mammalian hormones. There are studies that show that components in flaxseed inhibit growth of breast tumors.[273] Some studies show a lower incidence of breast cancer among people who eat more lignan containing foods. Flaxseed has actually been shown to reduce growth of breast cancer cells in a small placebo controlled study.[274] In animal studies, lignans have inhibited the growth of the breast tumors.[275]

---

[273] McCann SE et al. Sep 2004 *Int J Cancer* "Dietary lignan intakes and risk of pre- and postmenopausal breast cancer".

[274] Thompson LU et al. 2005 *Clin Cancer Res* "Dietary flaxseed alters tumor biological markers in postmenopausal breast cancer".

[275] Thompson LU et al Jun 1996 *Carcinogenesis* "Flaxseed and its lignin and oil components reduce mammary tumor growth at late stage of carcinogenesis".

According to Dr. Bob Arnot, flaxseed is best ground and you can eat up to 25 grams per day. Two tablespoons sprinkled on applesauce, yogurt, and cereal throughout the day will give you 3.2 g of omega-3. This will be enough to balance out one snack of eating nuts or one meal of eating meat. You may even find flaxseed in some bread or crackers, but this will not contribute enough to balance out omega-6.

I tried supplementing with two tablespoons of flaxseed each morning along with my protein shake. After a week of doing this, every day, I had some significant side effects including swollen and tender breasts and a headache. It is important to be aware that flaxseed has estrogenic properties, which you will want to be avoiding if you are detoxing estrogen. Also, it is well-known that flaxseed may be difficult for some people to digest. Chia seeds do not have any phytoestrogens, so that is my seed of choice right now.

There are three different types of omega-3 fatty acids. One is EPA (eicosapenaenoic acid). The second is DHA (docosahexaenoic acid). These first two have the most research to back up their health benefits and are typically derived from fish. The third is ALA (alpha-linolenic acid). ALA cannot be made in the body and flaxseed is the best source of ALA. In cellular studies, ALA plays a role of reducing inflammation. It has been directly linked with inhibiting breast cancer growth. ALA has to be converted to EPA and DHA to be helpful. Supposedly, only about 2 to 10% of the flaxseed we ingest actually gets converted to EPA and DHA, but flaxseed has still proven its benefits when it comes to breast cancer.

The four nuts with the fewest calories and lower fat content are almonds, cashews, macadamia and Brazil nuts. These would be good options for a snack or salad topping. Nuts can be very expensive however, so they do not need to be a mainstay in your diet.

Nuts that have been heat processed may contain more omega-6 and less nutrients, so it is a good idea to avoid them. The highest protein

216

nut appears to be Brazil nuts. You only need to eat six nuts to get 4g of protein. Cashews and Brazil nuts seem to be the best option for people with hypothyroid, as some nuts can also be goitrogenic (inhibit the production of thyroid hormones). Coconut has become a popular choice for the gluten free diet or in baking. Coconut does not have any omega-3, is low in omega-6, but has some saturated fat. It is important to not overdo it with nuts. If you do eat nuts, a small handful is plenty and it will be important to eat seeds, fish or a fish oil supplement to balance them out.

Not only can fat ratios be high in nuts, but one type of nut is known for contamination. Dr. Joseph Mercola says this about peanuts:

"most peanuts are very susceptible to contamination by aflatoxin, a carcinogenic mold spore, and so you should seek to restrict peanut butter (and any type of peanut product) consumption to Valencia peanuts only. This species grows in dry climates, which seriously restricts the growth of aflatoxin. Fortunately, Arrowhead Mills Organic Peanut Butter (which you can find in many stores now) meets both qualifications."

Peanut butter is typically used as a good source of protein in many diets. It is important to make sure the peanuts you are eating are not grown with pesticides and that it is eaten in moderation. Sunflower butter is newer alternative to peanut butter, but it is very high in omega-6. Cashew butter appears to be the best alternative with low PUFAs and lower saturated fat to monounsaturated fat ratio.

Again, if you are eating nuts, you will need to take omega-3 supplements if you don't like to eat fish or seeds. You may be able to get

FAT CONTENT IN NUTS AND SEEDS

Nut or seed 1 oz.	# of Nuts	Omega-6	Omega-3	Saturated Fat
Chia Seed	1oz	2.15g	6.51g	1g
Flaxseed	1oz	2.19g	8.46g	1g
Almonds	23	4.3g	2.226mg	1g
Brazil Nuts	6	7.63g	6.7mg	4g
Walnuts	14 halves	14.13g	3.39g	1.5g
Cashews	18	2.89g	.59mg	3g
Macadamia	11	462mg	76mg	3.5g
Peanuts	1 oz.	4g	0	2g
Pecans	19 halves	7.65g	366mg	2g
Pine Nuts	165	12.47g	4.45mg	1.5g
Pistachios	49	5.06g	94mg	1.5g
Coconut dried		252mg	0	8-16.22g

some omega-3 from seaweed. You would need to ingest high amounts on a daily basis because 100g of seaweed provides only 100mg of EPA. The best things to do are eat organic meat and dairy, keep nuts to a minimum, use coconut and olive oils and then add 6oz of fish a couple times per week, along with some flaxseed. This will enable you to achieve a diet with small quantities of omega-6, chemical trans fats and hormone laced saturated fat and increased omega-3.

Soy (Phytoestrogens)

Because of its low cost and healthy reputation, one of the most commonly used phytoestrogen today is soy, derived from the soybean. Many foods contain high levels of this phytoestrogen. It's in everything from mayonnaise, salad dressing, bread, crackers, protein powders, protein bars, supplements, animal feed and skincare products.

Soy contains a unique source of isoflavones which are compounds that bind to estrogen receptors and exhibit weak estrogen-like effects under certain conditions. When binding to estrogen receptors, isoflavones can either block human estrogen from attaching to those receptors (the reason why it decreases breast cancer risk) or at concentrated levels can stimulate the receptor in the same way estrogen does.

Companies jumped on the soy band-wagon when a study came out in 1991 that determined soy was beneficial for prevention of breast cancer.[276] Many population studies since have shown that ingestion of soy in Asian countries is linked to decreased breast cancer risk of up to 77%.[277] [278]

More recently, there has been controversy with the theory that soy lowers breast cancer risk. Human population studies on soy intake in the US, though small and short duration, show no link to breast cancer at all. Newer cellular and rodent studies are showing that isoflavones may actually stimulate breast cancer cells.

What is not considered in these studies is the effect of various types of soy foods as well as soy intake through the skin. Many studies in the US are utilizing concentrated soy isoflavones instead of non-GMO, fermented soy foods. 93% of soy in the US is GMO. Studies showing a reduced risk of breast cancer are all based on the Asian population's diet, not the US GMO soy diet. The main issue with population studies is that they do not take into account the types of soy being ingested or amount of soy being passed through meats via animal feed, soybean oils in condiments and other processed soy here in the US. Certainly,

---

[276] Lee HP et al. 1991 *Lancet* "Dietary effects on breast-cancer risk in Singapore".
[277] Messina MJ and Wood C 2008 *Nutritional Journal* "Soy isoflavones, estrogen therapy, and breast cancer risk: analysis and commentary."
[278] Wada K et al. Aug 2013 *Int J Cancer* "Soy isoflavone intake and breast cancer risk in Japan: from the Takayama study".

these are not the type of soy foods that are being ingested in Asian studies that show decreased risk. Fermented soy such as miso or tempeh is an entirely different ball game.

Due to added soy in many condiments and cosmetic products, we may be overdosing on a type of soy that is not good for us (unfermented and GMO), without even realizing it. It would be difficult to have a control in a US study because soy exists in some manner in most of our foods and cosmetics. There is no real control, except for those of us avoiding soy due to allergies or breast cancer prevention. Perhaps, if the various types of soy were isolated out, there may be different results.

Suffice to say, there have been mountains of studies in regards to soy, and hence various theories about its use have evolved. Dr. Bob Arnot teaches in his book, that it is healthy to eat soy as long as it is full of genistein. This is one of soy's main circulating isoflavones and is the most studied isoflavone that protects against breast cancer. He recommends 40 to 60 mg per day.

However, as Dr. Joseph Mercola points out, it is very difficult to count how much genistein you are getting each day. Along with many cellular studies, a 2004 rodent study showed ingesting high amounts of genistein could actually *increase* breast cancer tumor growth, specifically if it is processed soy.[279] Since most of the soy grown in the US is genetically modified, this means there are pesticides in the food. This may be another reason why rodent studies are showing growth in breast cancer tumors. Processed soy powder has higher concentrations of genistein and is not recommended by oncologists, especially if you are taking tamoxifen. Genistein has been shown to decrease tamoxifen's effect in some studies.

The *Mayo Clinic Breast Cancer Book* authors reviewed studies on soy

---

[279] Allred CD et al. Sep 2004 *Carcinogenesis* "Soy processing influences growth of estrogen-dependent breast cancer tumors".

and determined that most studies have not found that high soy intake cuts breast cancer risk. They also found that if you have thyroid issues, soy can negatively affect your thyroid. Yes, it is another goitrogen.

A doctor by the name of Dr. Richard Brouse of Shaklee endorses soy in Shaklee's supplement products because of the research they have performed over time. He has multiple recommendations when purchasing soy, which I found interesting. Here they are:

- The beans must be organic and not genetically engineered
- Each batch must be checked to confirm that it contains the 9 essential amino acids
- The crushed soy flakes must be water washed, not alcohol washed in the manufacturing process
- The anti-thyroid/anti-growth substance must be removed
- The process must be without heat
- The soy isolate must have calcium added to keep it a neutral grain

It doesn't sound easy to find a soy product you would want to use. From the research that I have found, it seems perfectly acceptable to eat fermented non-GMO soy in small amounts, but avoid all processed or GMO soy, which is what I do. Unfortunately, this means I have to read a lot of labels.

Whichever decision you make in regards to soy, you either have to do research on all your soy products, or you would have to avoid it completely, which in itself is almost impossible. We are being flooded with soy in most condiments and packaged products. I didn't realize how ubiquitous soy was until I started investigating.

As you can see from this next table, soy and flaxseed have the most phytoestrogen content of all the foods measured. The next few items down on the list are all soy products, so you can see how important it is to be aware how much soy and flaxseed you are digesting when it comes to your hormonal health. Too much may not be a good thing.

Foods High in Phytoestrogens Content

The total phytoestrogen content is the sum of isoflavones (genistein, daidzein, glycitein, formononetin), lignans (secoisolariciresinol, matairesinol, pinoresinol, lariciresinol), and coumestan (coumestrol). (**1 µg = 0.000001 g**) Data from Table 1 from www.dietaryfiber.com

Phytoestrogen food sources	Phytoestrogens content (µg/100g)
Flaxseed	379380
Soybeans	103920
Soy nuts	68730.8
Tofu	27150.1
Tempeh	18307.9
Miso paste	11197.3
Soy yogurt	10275
Soy protein powder	8840.7
Sesame seed	8008.1
Flax bread	7540
Multigrain bread	4798.7
Soy milk	2957.2
Hummus	993
Garlic	603.6
Mung bean sprouts	495.1
Dried apricots	444.5
Alfalfa sprouts	441.4
Pistachios	382.5
Dried dates	329.5
Sunflower seed	216
Chestnuts	210.2
Olive oil	180.7
Almonds	131.1
Cashews	121.9
Green bean	105.8

EAT 6: HIGH FIBER GRAINS; **Avoid Gluten, Sugar, Starch, Alcohol and Caffeine**

Fiber

A high fiber diet helps to move the bowels, which in turn moves the bad estrogens out of the body. It is important to rid the body of the bad estrogens or they will be re-absorbed into the system.

The best way to get fiber into your diet is with vegetables like Brussels sprouts, turnips and cabbage. A compound known as Diindolylmethane (DIM), as discussed in Step S, is found in cruciferous vegetables like broccoli sprouts and cabbage, and is believed to be helpful in fending off hormone fueled cancers. It stimulates production of enzymes in the liver that help break down chemicals and excess hormones. According to a June 2012 issue of *Natural Health Magazine*, a study from the University of Illinois suggests that as little as three to five servings of broccoli per week can have an anti-cancer effect.

Other high fiber foods are non-GMO grains. It is good to find breads with grains such as flaxseeds, millet and quinoa instead of rice, potatoes and wheat.

Both my son and my husband are gluten intolerant, so finding good fiber that has low sugar can be even more of a challenge. I went looking for gluten free, oat bran cereal instead of rice and corn cereals. I started substituting potatoes and rice with millet, quinoa and buckwheat.

I also started utilizing beans for increased fiber. Kidney, pinto, Lima, butter, black and navy beans are all excellent options. Unfortunately, some beans can be difficult to digest, so they are best eaten with an enzyme tablet.

Some people have a hard time digesting fiber in general. According to Dr. Natasha Campbell-McBride, fiber is not healthy for the gut if the stomach is not in good shape. She describes in full detail on Dr. Joseph Mercola's website what happens in the gut from infancy to adulthood and why some people have problems like gluten intolerance.

Our family tried Dr. Campbell-McBride's GAPS diet and loved some of the recipes. My child was actually cured from gluten intolerance after putting him on this diet, along with taking enzymes and probiotics. Anyway, if you are having trouble digesting certain foods, and are currently doing estrogen detox, wait to go on this diet because it limits your fiber intake. Taking some good probiotics with any of the foods you eat, along with some fiber will keep things moving along.

Another diet we are now trying is the Paleo diet. It is more of a way of life because all natural ingredients are used. Like the GAPS diet, it eliminates all grains and encourages organic meats and lots of vegetables and fruit. I eat a salad every day for lunch to make sure I have adequate fiber intake with this diet. Children have a tough time not eating carbohydrates on the Paleo diet, so you can still make corn and quinoa noodles and utilize other fibrous grains.

Sugar

I think it is safe to say that as a society, we are addicted to sugar and starches. Everywhere we go, in every processed food we eat, there are sugars, and starches. Some, in an effort to reduce fats in their diet, intake more sugar in carbohydrates. If you take a peek at the next chart, you can see how much sugar consumption has increased over time in our society.

Sugar is an addiction! Even when we are on a strict diet, there's always this little craving for sugar whether it be for a piece of chocolate, or a bite of a donut. Although we have the freedom to do what we want with our bodies, we become enslaved by these addictions...adding them to our way of everyday life.

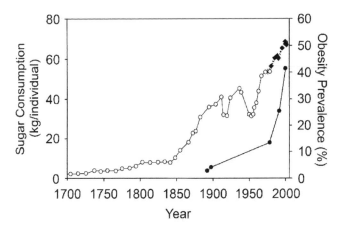

Source: Johnson RJ, et al. Potential role of sugar (fructose) in the epidemic of hypertension, obesity and the metabolic syndrome, diabetes, kidney disease, and cardiovascular disease. The American Journal Of Clinical Nutrition, 2007.

The problem with this addiction is both sugar and starch increase insulin. Insulin increases estrogen, along with a whole host of other bad effects. Sugar also raises uric acid, which in high amounts in the blood is known to cause gout, diabetes or even kidney stones. Here is what Dr. Joseph Mercola says about fructose and uric acid:

"It's been known that meats and purine rich foods can raise uric acid, but it turns out that one of the most potent ways to raise uric acid is by consuming large amounts of fructose! *You probably already know fructose is a sugar, but you may not realize is that it's distinctly different from other sugars, as it's metabolized in your body through very specific pathways that differ from those of glucose. Uric acid is a byproduct of* <u>fructose metabolism</u>. *In fact, fructose typically generates uric acid within minutes of ingestion."[280]*

---

[280] Dr. Joseph Mercola Oct 13, 2009 http://articles.<u>mercola.com</u> "Artificial Sweeteners –More Dangerous Than You Ever Imagined".

You can see that fructose is not good to digest in high amounts. If you want to know how bad off your fructose intake is, you can test your uric acid. A simple 24-hour urine collection test and you will find out how you fair! You can order a kit online or you can order it through your doctor. This is will also tell you if you may be prone to gout, kidney stones or other problems.

There is also a glucose blood test available called HbA1c. This will give you your long term (three month) average of glucose. Most of us already know we eat too much sugar and a test is not really necessary, unless you are diabetic, borderline diabetic or have a history of low blood sugar.

It is important to know the difference between all the "oses" when selecting which sweetener you will use. Glucose is needed by all living things to produce energy. Sucrose is table sugar which is 50% glucose and 50% fructose. Fructose is processed by the body differently than high amounts of glucose. Some doctors believe fructose can be poison to the body. High fructose corn syrup is 45 to 55% fructose. High fructose corn syrup has been used extensively in foods in the US since the 1970s, since it is less expensive and less of it is needed to acquire the same sweetness as sugar. Anytime you see "corn syrup" on the label, you are looking at fructose. You would need to eliminate sugar and corn syrup from the diet in order to reduce fructose intake.

Eliminating or significantly decreasing fructose and glucose can speed your path to prevention or recovery. Sugar is how cancer cells survive. Studies prove that removing cancer's source of sugar, shrinks tumors and that too much sugar may impact the future outcome of breast cancer patients.[281] [282]To stop eating sugar can be as difficult as fasting. It takes a strong will to overcome addictions and this one is not easy.

---

[281] Monzavi-Karbassi B et al. Sep 2010 *Int J Oncol* Fructose consumption may worsen the condition of breast cancer patients".
[282] Board M et al. Aug 1995 *Cancer Res* "High Km glucose-phosphorylating (glucokinase) activities in a range of tumor cell lines and inhibition of rates of tumor growth by the specific enzyme inhibitor mannoheptulose".

Sugars have similar or worse addictive tendencies than morphine or heroin. I found what Dr. Joseph Mercola says to be interesting:

"Sugar actually makes you eat more sugar. Eating it triggers the production of your brain's natural opioids -- a key factor in addiction. Your brain essentially becomes addicted to the sugar-induced opioid release, not unlike addictions to morphine or heroin. The more you eat, the more you crave. This vicious cycle underlies much the overconsumption of sugar today."[283]

There are some things you can use in moderation while you get over your addiction. As time goes on, you'll want to have a goal to only get your fructose from fruit. Even fruit should be limited. Dr. Joseph Mercola has created a handy table that shows you how much fructose is in fruit. You can find it here: http://articles.mercola.com/sites/articles/archive/2010/03/13/richard-johnson-interview.aspx. Limes, lemons, prunes and apricots have the lowest levels of fructose. Dried apricots and figs, mangos, grapes and raisins have the highest levels of fructose.

Having a plan to allow some sweets into your diet is a good idea to help get over sugar addiction. I typically substitute sweets with a slightly sweet drink such as green tea with honey. Green tea may be helpful in preventing breast cancer at the same time. There was a large study of women who drank green tea regularly that found they had a moderately lower risk of breast cancer.[284] *The Mayo Clinic Breast Cancer Book* says the scientific studies are mixed as to whether green tea is beneficial for protecting against breast cancer, but certainly one cup per day won't hurt you. Large quantities could interfere with chemotherapy medications, so be aware of that.

---

[283] Dr. Joseph Mercola Mar 2010 http://articles.mercola.com "Sugar: Is This Common Food Ingredient as Addictive as Cocaine?"
[284] Shrubsole MJ et al. Feb 2009 *J Nutrition* "Drinking green tea modestly reduces breast cancer risk".

Organic cane sugar and organic honey are good options for real sweeteners. Organic or all natural honey is known to be a prebiotic. Prebiotics are good bacteria that will grow in your digestive tract and can aid in digestion. Both can be very high in fructose though, so should be used in very small amounts. I use a teaspoon measuring spoon when using honey.

Stevia and xylitol are other replacements for sugar than can be used. Stevia powder is a little bitter, but is a good alternative for cutting out half the sugar in baking. Flavored liquid stevia is a tasty alternative for coffee or tea. We found that Truvia® a form of stevia, also tastes pretty good. Buying pure glucose (dextrose) is an even better option.

There are many sugar substitutes that are approved by the FDA for use. I could not find any research linking any of them directly to breast cancer in humans. However, there is some research linking them to other cancers in cells and mice (such as bladder cancer). The following are FDA approved sugar substitutes, some of which have been linked to some cancers:

Aspartame (Equal®, Nutrasweet®, Canderel® and AminoSweet®)
Sucralose (Splenda®)
Acesulfame K (Sunett®, Sweet One®)
Saccharine (Sweet'N Low®, Sugar Twin®)

As long as you are not using these artificial sweeteners extensively for long periods of time, there does not seem to be much health risk associated with using them. Some people report reactions to aspartame like headaches and dizziness. Also, it is a known fact that aspartame can turn into formaldehyde in the body. Formaldehyde is a known carcinogen by the EPA. So, knowing this, it may be a good idea to avoid aspartame.[285]

---

[285] Kirtida R Tandel 2011 *J Pharmacol Pharmacother* "Sugar substitutes: Health controversy over perceived benefits".

Starch and Gluten

It is important to know that starches are quickly transformed into sugar in the body, unless they are whole grain. You may have noticed that more companies are offering various and interesting grains in their ingredients. This trend is for a reason. Regular old wheat is getting the boot. Diabetes is on the rise along with people becoming intolerant to gluten. There are three changes over the past 50 years that have occurred in wheat that is most likely causing this intolerance. According to Dr. Mark Hyman the following items are in our bread:

1. A super starch called amylopectin A
2. Super gluten which is super inflammatory
3. A super drug that causes you to crave more bread

Dr. Hyman explains: *"What we grow now is dwarf wheat which is the product of genetic manipulation and hybridization that created short stubby, hardy, high yielding wheat plants with much higher amounts of starch and gluten and many more chromosomes coding for all sorts of new odd proteins. The man who engineered this modern wheat won the Nobel Prize – it promised to feed millions of starving around the world. Well, it has, and it has made them fat and sick."*[286]

White bread, even wheat bread or any bread labeled "whole grain" is really not the same as it used to be. Unless you can verify that the grain is whole grain wheat, stay away from it. Usually, if a product is labeled with health claims on the label, it is hiding something. It will make your sugar levels spike. I notice that every time I eat a sandwich with regular bread, I feel really tired afterwards. Food is supposed to be energy building, not depleting!

Starches to stay away from because they convert to sugar quickly are: potatoes, French fries, white rice, white bread, regular wheat bread. Sweet potatoes or brown rice are better but still convert to insulin fairly

---

[286] http://drhyman.com/blog/2012/2/13/three-hidden-ways-wheat-makes-you-fat/

quickly. Keep in mind that many gluten free breads have potato starches or rice in them which comes with an increase in insulin.

The following types of grains are slower to digest and less likely to convert to sugar: millet, quinoa and buckwheat. Quinoa is a favorite side for dinnertime as long as it is rinsed ahead of time. Buckwheat is a good hot cereal for breakfast. For bread, you may need to do some searching to find one with real whole grain, natural, organic, bromine free and pesticide free. Our family typically eats gluten free breads. One of our favorite is millet and zucchini bread made in Florida by DeLand Bakery. We can only find it at a local health food store, but it can be special ordered online at www.delandbakery.com. Keep in mind that millet is considered a goitrogen, which interferes with iodine uptake in your thyroid and may lead to goiter (enlarged thyroid). If you have hypothyroid, millet may not be good idea for you. The best bread to buy if you are not gluten intolerant by now is a real whole grain bread.

When I started evaluating my sugar intake, I was amazed at how much sugar I manage to sneak into my diet through fruit, carbohydrates and drinks without realizing it. Vitamin powder drinks, whey protein drinks, honey in tea and it all adds up to a lot more sugar than I should be eating. Dr. Joseph Mercola recommends not going above 25 grams of sugar per day. In order to achieve this, I had to use a teaspoon measurer when using any sweeteners. Measuring sweeteners helps keeps sugar under control and it's not *too* excruciating.

Alcohol and Coffee

Besides sugar as a food habit and addiction, some of us have drink addictions to coffee or alcoholic beverages. Unfortunately, alcohol is significantly linked to increased risk of breast cancer and caffeine may also have an association with it. Keeping caffeine and alcohol down to one drink per day...or none at all is probably a good idea.

Both the natural and medical communities agree that increased alcohol consumption directly correlates to a higher risk of developing breast cancer if you drink two or more drinks per day, and in some cases, just three or more per week. What is the reason? According to The Breast Cancer Prevention Institute Online Booklet, drinking alcohol increases breast cancer risk because of its effect on the liver. The liver is where estrogen is metabolized and when it is impaired by alcohol, it stores higher amounts, which in turn stimulates the breast.

The Willett study in 1987 showed that women who drank 5 to 14g (one drink) of alcohol per day had an increased relative risk of 30%. Those who drank 15g or more (one or more drinks) of alcohol per day had a 150% increased risk of breast cancer.[287] Many other studies have had similar results as the Willett study. Interestingly, if Premarin was added to the mix of two drinks per day, breast cancer risk was higher at 80%.[288]

Another thing that alcohol does is release iron from its bound proteins in breast tissue. Free iron can cause inflammation at high amounts and is found in breast cancer patients.

If you quit drinking, will it significantly decrease your chances of getting breast cancer? Well, lower alcohol consumption has shown to decrease your risk by 20% according to the Mayo Clinic. It sounds like a good idea

---

[287] Willett WC et al May 1987 *N Engl J Med* "Moderate alcohol consumption and the risk of breast cancer".
[288] Dorgan JF et al. May 2001 *J Natl Cancer Inst* "Serum hormones and the alcohol-breast cancer association in postmenopausal women".

to keep alcohol to one drink or less per day. In case you want to be precise, one drink equals 12 ounces of beer, 5 ounces of wine or 1.5 ounces of 80 proof distilled liquor.

There is mixed evidence regarding coffee and caffeine increasing or decreasing risk. Most studies indicate no significant risk for breast cancer and many show a decreased risk. It is evident from these studies that genes are a key determining factor.[289] It seems the actual coffee bean itself can lower your risk if separated out from caffeine.[290] The risk of breast cancer while drinking coffee shows up significantly with women already diagnosed with breast cancer. Patients who drank three or more cups per day had a lower survival rate.[291]

Interestingly, my doctor informed me that a breast thermography test can be done one or two hours after drinking a cup of coffee to see how the body reacts to the coffee. According to my doctor, some people have a better vascular pattern after one cup of coffee. If you are addicted to that morning cup of coffee, you could reduce your caffeine by cutting your usual brew with increasing amounts of decaffeinated coffee over time. Caffeinated sodas are just not a good idea due to added sugar, so it's a good idea to limit them to special occasions.

Note on Alkaline Foods

After reading several articles about alkaline foods and their effect on cancers, I have come to the conclusion that there is nothing wrong with eating alkaline foods. It certainly will not harm you. Some scientists say that alkaline foods do not turn into alkaline blood or tissue in your body. Most articles say that cancer can indeed grow in an alkaline environment. The tests performed on cancer in the labs use an alkaline

---

[289] Jiang W et al. Jun 2013 *Gynecol Oncol* "Coffee and caffeine intake and breast cancer risk: An updated dose-response meta-analysis of 37 published studies".

[290] Lowcock EC et al. 2013 *Nutr Cancer* "High Coffee intake, but not caffeine, is associated with reduced estrogen receptor negative and postmenopausal breast cancer risk with no effect modification by CYP1A2genotype".

[291] Lehrer S et al. Mar 2013 J *Caffeine Res Coffee* Consumption Associated with Increased Mortality of Women with Breast Cancer".

environment to grow cancer, after all. All articles concur that cancer growth does slow down at extreme alkaline levels due to lack of oxygen.

Regardless, foods that are alkaline are good for your body. If you look up a list of alkaline foods, you will find that some lists differ in opinion about what is alkaline and what is not. Alkaline recommendations for meat, vegetables, fish, milk, sweets and grain are similar to the recommendations for food to eat in this section anyway. They focus on eating more fruit and vegetables and less grain, milk, sweets and meat.

Either way, testing your pH or not, eating good foods may help prevent cancer. I wouldn't get too caught up in the disagreement about which foods are alkaline and which are acidic. Stay focused on low sugar, low carb and pesticide free! Full lists of acid vs. alkaline foods are at www.eatforlife.org if you want to try the alkaline route.

Healthy Choices for Fast Paced Society

Eating healthily 100% of the time is next to impossible and aiming to be a perfect eater, spells failure. In today's society there are too many food obstacles, so we have to be realistic. That's why I try to stick to a healthy diet 80 to 90% of the time. If you calculate this out for three meals a day, seven days a week, that leaves you with at least two meals where you can go off diet. I try to save these meals for the end of the week when I am tired and apt to grab fast food or attend social activities with friends. At home, during the week I plan meals, so I don't have to wait till last minute to cook. See Chapter 17 for more ideas on eating well at home.

Still, there are things you can do to try to stay on the diet even outside the home. First, you can keep healthy snacks in the car. These may include seaweed snacks, seeds, nuts, veggies, fruit or beet chips. When we are out and about and starving, these can hold us over until we can get home. If you travel a lot like me, this is a life safer.

Second, you can make a list of all the organic, natural restaurants or fast food places in the area and keep that list in the car. If you need to stop to eat, it will give you good choices without having to think. Consumer Reports did an analysis on fast food places to determine which ones have hormone free meat. There were two restaurants on the list. You can look those up as part of your healthy eating choices. There is definitely a trend of moving toward healthier hormone free meat at restaurants. Though eating at a fast food place may not be top choice, at least we know there are better alternatives. If you have a little more time, kabob restaurants may be a good idea. I spoke to the owners of one of these restaurants in the area and he explained that due to their religious traditions, their meats are raised without GMOs or pesticides.

Thirdly, before attending an event, I ask if there is anything I can bring. I always offer to bring the vegetables. I find that many parties are lacking vegetables and a veggie tray or salad is an easy dish to put together. This gives me a healthy side to munch on to keep me from filling up on other stuff.

Chapter 15

E is for ERADICATE EXTERNAL PROESTROS

This second Step E is about limiting proestros that get into our bodies from our outside environment. These external proestros are found in products that we use on a daily basis, but are also found in the air we breathe, the water we drink, and the products we touch.

Many natural environmental substances and man-made chemicals act as proestros and come in several forms. They may enter our body through our skin, lungs or mouth. It seems we can't win. Every time we turn around, there is some new substance with estrogenic properties in it. In the Silent Spring Institute report detailing 216 common chemicals found to cause breast tumors in animals, 73 of these are present in consumer products or food. 35 are air pollutants and 25 are associated with occupational exposures. The Silent Spring Institute database includes references to 900 studies. These study results appeared in the June 2007 issue of the American Cancer Society's journal "*Cancer*". A complete database of environmental and dietary factors and their effects on breast cancer can be found on www.Silentspring.org. Just search for "database".

It is no wonder that the cause of breast cancer cannot be targeted to one thing. There are so many chemicals in our environment that contribute to it. But preventing breast cancer does not have to be overwhelming because many of these can be avoided simultaneously. Since there is an abundance of external proestros, the focus in this book will discuss the most common ones that surround us, the ones we have control of and those that have significant scientific data to support a possible breast cancer influence.

One of the ways we can avoid these chemicals is by checking the labels on products that we use regularly. I was surprised at all the old lotions, cleaners and pans I was hoarding that had proestros in them. Some products were over 25 years old! Getting rid of proestro-laden products becomes an easy decision once we learn how bad they are for the body. These are chemicals and substances we can't even see or taste, yet our bodies are fighting a war against them!

External proestros have some of the highest relative risks for breast cancer. That is why it is imperative to eradicate these out of your life. For simplification, I have narrowed down 20 external proestros into seven categories. This section will discuss what they are, where you can find them, how they are linked to breast cancer, as well as suggestions for avoiding them. Really, all you need is the reference chart below so you can see which ones are affecting you and what healthier choices you can make. If you want to understand more about each one, read this entire section.

Avoid External Proestros

External Proestro	How Exposed	Healthy options	Don'ts
Aluminum	*Ingested-* transdermal, alcohol, wine aluminum cookware, drinking water, food additives, drinking bottles, antacids, *Transdermal-* vaccines, deodorant	Ceramic or glass cookware and drinking bottles, filter your water, limit vaccines, buy aluminum free deodorant	Do not drink alcohol or wine regularly, do not take antacids regularly

External Proestro	How Exposed	Healthy options	Don'ts
Arsenic	*Ingested*- meat, vegetables from arsenic residues in soil and animal feed, ground water *Inhaled* – ambient air, treated wood prior to 2002, herbicides	Research food manufacturer arsenic content, rinse vegetables, rice and fruit, filter your water	Don't eat rice more than once per week, do not sand pressure treated wood, do not live near a golf course or sod farm that uses arsenical herbicides
Bisphenol (BPA)	*Ingested* - Plastic food containers, plastic wrap, canned food, garden hoses, resin cavity fillings *Transdermal* - receipts	Glass storage, email receipts glass jar food, foil and wax paper wrapped foods	Do not drink from garden hoses, limit canned food
Cleaning Solvents	*Inhaled* – air freshener, dish soap, laundry detergent, furniture polish, mold cleaner	Baking soda, Vinegar, hydrogen peroxide, essential oils, fragrance free detergent	Do not use fragrance oils or air fresheners

External Proestro	How Exposed	Healthy options	Don'ts
Copper	*Ingested* - fungicides, wood preservative, copper plumbing supply pipes, vitamin supplements, copper cookware	Filter your water, check your supplements for copper, use ceramic and glass cookware	Don't use fungicides, don't use copper cookware, don't sand pressure treated wood
Flame Retardant	*Transdermal* -cell phones, alarm clocks, computers, *Inhaled* - couch cushions, carpet padding, mattresses, curtains, appliances, toner cartridges	Dust often with a wet rag, use a HEPA vacuum, buy products w/o flame retardants, buy wool, cotton, and down, wear a mask when working with insulation, wash hands after handling electrical equipment, cover couches	Do not change upholstery yourself at your home
Lead	*Inhaled and ingestion* - lead paint, lead supply plumbing or solder, industrial workplace	Filter water, have house tested for lead paint	Do not sand lead paint, do not work near lead based products.

External Proestro	How Exposed	Healthy options	Don'ts
Mercury	*Ingested* – fish, antiseptics, laxatives, metal filings *Transdermal*- flu vaccine *Inhaled*- charcoal plant, fluorescent bulbs if broken, mascara	Limit fish and choose fish with lower mercury levels. Take vitamin D and C daily, buy LED light bulbs, replace metal fillings with resin	Do not get metal fillings or the flu vaccine, do not live near a charcoal plant, do not break fluorescent light bulbs containing mercury
Organo-chlorine Pesticides	Herbicides and insecticides	Use diatomaceous earth for insect control, make home-made bug traps	Don't use pesticides
Parabens	*Ingested*- processed foods *Transdermal*- cosmetics, spermicides, hair care, all personal care products	Use paraben free personal care products: lotion, shampoo, conditioner, soap, lipstick, cosmetics	Don't use spermicides regularly

External Proestro	How Exposed	Healthy options	Don'ts
Perfluorin ated Com-pounds i.e. PFCs, PFOA	*Ingested-* water, Teflon cookware, microwave popcorn *Transdermal-* shampoo *Inhaled* – industrial waste, Scotchguard, plastic shower curtains	Filter your water, use a popcorn machine, ceramic cookware, buy PFOA free products	Don't use Teflon pans, *Scotchguard* or floor wax, Don't eat bagged microwave popcorn
Phthalates	*Ingested-* plastic food wrapping, medication, drinking water. *Inhaled* – cleaning products, shower curtain, new car, PVC flooring, perfume, nail polish, hair spray *Transdermal* – lotion, shampoo, make-up, deodorant	Buy cheese wrapped in foil or wax paper. American cheese plastic is ok. Check and change Rx for phthalates, filter your water, use vinegar, baking soda and Borax for cleaning, buy used cars or phthalate free, buy personal care products without phthalates	Don't buy pre-made cleaners, don't buy cheese wrapped in plastic

240

External Proestro	How Exposed	Healthy options	Don'ts
Polycyclic aromatic Hydrocarbons (PAH)	*Inhaled* - Burning of coal, wood, gas, oil, garbage, fat, incense or tobacco, cigarette smoke, vehicle emissions, asphalt paving, camp fires, wood stoves *Transdermal* - tattoos	Well vented combustible appliances, recirculate air in car when driving behind trucks or old cars, use vapor cigarettes if you must smoke	Avoid getting tattoos, breathing in camp fire or stove exhaust, don't live near a coal plant, don't burn incense or smoke and avoid 2nd hand smoke, don't work at asphalt paving site, don't cook meat on a high flame

External Proestro	How Exposed	Healthy options	Don'ts
Radiation	*Transdermal-* X-rays, mammograms, airline check points, fluorescent light bulbs, wireless phones, cell phones, computers, smart meters, Wi-Fi, chargers, towers, kitchen appliances	Use thermography annually, use speaker phone, headset or blue tooth for cell phone, use battery alarm, unplug chargers, plug in when not home, buy computers with EMF reducer on cord (laptops have this), test house for high levels EMF if near a tower	Do not use fluorescent light bulbs, do not wear cell phone on the body, do not keep alarm or cell phone next to your bed, do not stand in front of the fridge, microwave or toaster oven for long periods, opt out of check points or get speed check if traveling regularly

Eradicate 1: BISPHENOLS

BPA, and BPS (bisphenols) are man-made plastic chemicals that are used in the manufacture of polycarbonate containers. These plastics leach into food or drinks from containers. If used in the microwave, BPA is released 55 times faster. There are more types of bisphenols than you could ever imagine. They range from bisphenol AB and AF to

242

bisphenol-Z. Bisphenol-A (BPA) was banned in Canada and banned in baby bottles in the US in 2012 because it mimics estrogen in the body and has been associated with increased risk for breast cancer, among other diseases.

The main means of exposure to BPA is by ingestion, but it can also be absorbed through the skin. Everyone is exposed to BPA at some level because it exists in many everyday products. A recent study found 88% of 2000 pregnant Canadian women had BPA in their bodies.[292] Another study by the CDC, the first using a human population as reference, showed that 92.6% of over 2500 Americans had BPA in their urine.[293] BPA has been found in milk of nursing mothers as well. This is an indication that fetuses and newborns are readily exposed to this chemical.

BPA is found in canned food, plastic food containers, plastic wrap, and garden hoses. I recently found out that BPA is in resin tooth fillings in your mouth! The resin is only about 1 to 5% BPA, but with all the media exposure, you would think the BPA would be removed! I guess I'd better not get any more cavities.

In July 2010, the Environmental Working Group (EWG) found high levels of BPA on 40% of thermal paper receipts (the kind that change color when you scratch them). In some cases, the amount of BPA measured was 1000 times greater than what was found in common food sources. Most research on BPA has focused on levels from ingested sources, but per Natural Health Magazine (July/August 2012), a study published in July 2011 found that BPA transfers readily from receipts and can penetrate the skin to such a depth that it can't be washed off. When at the check-out counter, I just ask the clerk to throw the receipt away or put it in the bag. More recently, there is an option for emailed receipts.

[292] Dr. Marisa Weiss Sep 2014 www.breastcancer.org "An Update on BPA".
[293] Calafat AM, Ye X et al. 2008 *Environ Health Perspect* "Exposure of the U.S. population to bisphenol A and 4-tertiary-octylphenol 2003-2004."

BPA has been known to mimic estrogen since the 1930s. In fact, they used it as a hormone replacement for women and an artificial estrogen to fatten poultry and cattle. Bayer and General Electric started using it in plastics in the 1940s.

Animal and cellular studies have linked BPA exposure to breast, brain, prostate cancer, heart disease as well as disorders of the nervous and immune systems. In regards to breast cancer, scientists have found in cellular studies that BPA can work with natural estrogen in the body to interfere with genes that stop cancer from growing.[294] Also, BPA was found to encourage growth of inflammatory breast cancer at BPA levels typically found in human blood, *regardless* of estrogen receptor-positive or negative test results. In this same study, BPA made inflammatory breast cancer cells resistant to treatment. In other words, BPA is stronger than the drugs we have available today to stop it.

BPA can also make more permanent changes in infants and children. Exposure at a young age made baby rats' mammary glands develop differently and increased the likelihood for them to develop breast cancer later in life. [295]This is why it was banned in infant and children's products in the US in 2012.

Breast cancer is not the only way BPA effects the hormonal system. BPA can harm development of ovaries and affect pregnancy outcome. A small study showed that the risk of miscarriage was 83% greater in women with high levels of BPA. BPA also affects men. New research shows BPA may be harmful to testicular function and may cause infertility. BPA is directly linked to a decrease in sperm count. Lastly,

---

[294] Lee HR, Hwang KA, et al May 2012 *Int J Mol Med* "Treatment with bisphenol A and methoxychlor results in the growth of human breast cancer cells and alteration of the expression of cell cycle-related genes, cyclin D1 and p21, via an estrogen receptor-dependent signaling pathway."

[295] Soto AM, Brisken C, et al June 2013 *J Mammary Gland Biol Neolasia* "Does cancer start in the womb? Altered mammary gland development and predisposition to breast cancer due to in utero exposure to endocrine disruptors."

recent studies show men with prostate cancer had much higher levels of BPA in their urine. You can see how detrimental this chemical can be to our hormonal system and it goes without saying, it would be wise to avoid BPA completely.

The policy makers in the US have invoked the *precautionary principle* for children in regards to BPA. This principle is used when there is plausible evidence to show cause and effect in animals. Regulators will advise caution when using products where the principle has been invoked. Based on this precautionary principle, the European Food Safety Authority has lowered the tolerable daily intake of BPA to 5 micrograms per kilogram of body weight, down from 50 mg/kg/d. The US limit remains at 50ug/kg body weight based on ingested amounts. There have been bills introduced in both the US House and Senate, but Congress and the FDA are very conservative about banning products. Scientists, including breast cancer oncologist Dr. Marisa Weiss, are concerned that at even low levels, BPA over the course of a lifetime can have a negative effect.

There have not been enough studies on other types of bisphenols, but Dr. Joseph Mercola cites studies on Bisphenol-S, the latest and greatest bisphenol, being used in the BPA free products. It seems that Bisphenol-S doesn't look better than the A kind. In fact, it could be worse. Dr. Marisa Weiss also warns that new alternative plastics are no safer than BPA and may be even less safe.[296]

The good news is that we can effectively eliminate most BPAs from ingestion. A study published in 2011 in *Environmental Health Perspectives,* found that people who consumed a fresh diet without BPAs for three days, dropped BPA levels by 66%. All you have to do is avoid using all plastic containers for food and drink storage as well as food pre-packaged in plastic. Canned foods are also lined with bisphenols, so avoiding canned food is a good idea as well. Some

---

[296] Dr. Marisa Weiss Sep 2014 www.breastcancer.org "An Update on BPA".

canned products are advertising BPA free, but who knows what bisphenol they used as a substitute.

Using all glass or ceramic jars, drinking bottles, food storage, mixing bowls and containers will get rid of most of your BPA exposure. Glass storage and drink containers are found in most stores, but I bought mine from *Costco*, www.DrMercola.com and www.amazon.com. Ceramic and stainless steel coffee mugs are a good option for hot/cold drinks. *Five Below* sells cups and mugs that are ceramic so you don't have to spend a lot of money to lower your body burden. Many foods are being sold in glass jars such as spaghetti sauce. Canning vegetables or soup broth in Mason jars is a good alternative if you have the time.

The BPA issue gives us another reason to try and eat mostly fresh food. If you do get canned foods, buy organic if possible, to minimize total chemical intake. Do not use plastic wrap while heating food. Do not microwave food in plastic containers. Get rid of plastic drinking cups. If you work at a store register using thermal receipts, wear non-vinyl gloves. Lastly, don't drink from outside hoses.

Eradicate 2: PHTHALATES

Phthalates are added to plastics such as polyvinyl chloride (PVC), to increase flexibility, transparency, and durability. When tested by the Centers for Disease Control and Prevention, most Americans were found to have multiple phthalates in their urine. [297] Phthalates are found in many sources that surround us. They are believed to be mostly ingested, but phthalates are easily released into the environment through the air and absorbed through the skin and lungs. We absorb them through personal care products. We ingest them through food wrappings and containers and medications. We inhale them through house building materials, cars and cleaning supplies. When these

---

[297] CDC July 2005 "Third National Report on Human Exposure to environmental Chemicals".

phthalate products are disposed of and released into the air and ground they can end up in drinking water.

Phthalates can be categorized into three groups based on their weight. The lower weight phthalates are the ones that are easily inhaled, absorbed and ingested. The higher weight phthalates are not as easily absorbed and are not considered hazardous. Also, it is well documented that phthalates can accumulate in the body, causing even small amounts to build up and interact with other chemicals, which has cumulative adverse effects.[298]

Rat studies have shown that when exposed to these lower weight phthalates, large amounts will change hormone levels and cause birth defects. Multiple human observational studies show an association between phthalate exposure and endocrine disruption leading to breast cancer.[299] A case control study in 2009 on healthy girls who started breast development before age 8, showed that they had increased levels of monomethyl phthalate (MMP).[300] A study in 2010 published in *Environmental Health Perspectives*, implicated exposure to diethyl phthalates (DEP) may be associated with increased risk of breast cancer.[301] DEP is found in high levels in personal care products, deodorants and perfumes. A study in 2013 linked phthalates and BPA with higher mammographic breast density.[302] As you already have seen, increased breast density is linked to increased risk of breast cancer.

---

[298] Waring, RH and Harris, RM *Cancer.org* 2011 "Endocrine disrupters – a threat to women's health?"

[299] Cancer.org May 2011 "Breast Cancer Risk Factors"

[300] Chou YY et al. Jan 2009 *J Pediatr Endocrinol Metab* "Phthalate exposure in girls during early puberty."

[301] Lopez-Carillo L, Herndandez-Ramirez RU et al. 2010 *Environmental Health Perspectives* "Exposure to phthalates and breast cancer risk in Northern Mexico."

[302] Sprague BL et al. May 2013 *Breast Cancer Res* "Circulating serum xenoestrogens and mammographic breast density."

Dermal exposures may contribute greatly to a woman's body burden of phthalates. Lower weight phthalates are found in most cosmetics and personal care products such as lotions and shampoos. Other personal care items with phthalates include eye shadow, moisturizer, nail polish, liquid soap, hair spray and perfume. Women have higher levels of phthalates because we use more personal care products.

Ingestion from wrappings or containers is another way phthalates make it into the body. Phthalate plasticizers are not chemically bound to PVC so they can easily leach and evaporate into food or the air from containers. This gives us another reason to buy alternatives to plastic storage containers. Plastic coatings on product containers leach into fatty foods such as milk, butter and meat and are therefore a major source of phthalates as well. In 1999, *Consumer Reports* analyzed fourteen brands of deli cheese wrapped in six types of plastic. A large amount of the phthalate DEHA was found in the cheeses stored in deli cling wrap. Interestingly, no migration was found in individually wrapped American cheese slices or cheddar laminated in foil wrap. Recycled delivery pizza boxes have also been found to contain phthalates.

Phthalates are also found in pharmaceutical coatings and can even be found in medications by leaching from plastic containers. A recent study found that urine concentrations of phthalates from pharmaceuticals can far exceed levels from other sources.[303] It would be prudent to find out if any prescriptions you are taking have phthalates in or on them.

Besides food and medications, phthalates can also be ingested from plastic toys. The US passed a law in 2009 to make it unlawful to manufacture, sell or distribute children's toys containing phthalates that can be put in the mouth. Most parents may be aware of this

---

[303] Hernandez-Diaz et al. Feb 2009 *Environ Health Perspect* "Medications as a Potential Source of Exposure to Phthalates in the U.S. Population."

change by now, but if not, it would be a good idea to throw out old plastic toys.

Home and car materials as well as cleaning products are yet another absorbed source of phthalates through inhalation and dermal exposure. Phthalates are found in your car, shower curtains, pesticides and cleaning supplies. We are surrounded by phthalates. Shower curtains are available without phthalates if you just check the label. You know that knew car smell we all love? That's phthalates we are inhaling and enjoying. The good news is that 17% of new cars are being manufactured without PVCs and phthalates and 60% without flame retardants such as perfluorinated compounds (PFCs). A 2008 Bulgarian study found higher dust concentration levels of low weight phthalates where furniture polishing agents are used.[304] For this reason, you may want to consider using basic cleaning supplies, such as vinegar, borax and baking soda.

The US is gradually replacing lower weight phthalates with higher weight phthalates. Europe has regulated phthalates, utilizing types that are not classified as hazardous (DINP and DIDP). Considered a low hazard, di (2-ethylhexyl phthalate (DEHP) and diisononyl phthalate (DIDP) have been phased out in Europe as of February 2015. The EPA has regulations in place for public drinking water. The maximum containment level is 6 ppb for public water systems. This does not protect private water systems, so having a good filter, if you have a well, is a good idea.

In order to lower our body burden of this toxin, we can take several steps. We can evaluate ingredients in our body lotions, deodorant, and make-up. We can avoid drinking out of or eating out of plastic containers. We can reduce eating canned food. We can utilize natural cleaners and read labels for household plastic items such as shower curtains.

---

[304] Kolarik B, Bornehag C et al. Aug 2008 *Atmospheric Environment* "The concentration of phthalates in settled dust in Bulgarian homes in relation to building characteristic and cleaning habits in the family."

Most plastic products have some type of chemical in them that is associated with breast cancer. This is why we need to try to work harder to protect our bodies. We may not be able to eradicate phthalates completely out of our products, but we can certainly lower it going into our body so we can process it out!

Eradicate 3: PARABENS

Parabens are a class of chemicals used as preservatives in processed foods, cosmetics and pharmaceuticals in order to extend their shelf-life. They are also in spermicides, hair care products, body lotions and cleansers. There are conflicting facts on parabens. Some studies and reviews have shown evidence of parabens acting as a weak estrogen. Some show no evidence that parabens act as an estrogen at all. The Environmental Working Group's (EWG) website evaluates products according to their toxicity. According to EWG, paraben is an ingredient that is considered toxic, has estrogenic affects and has been linked with breast cancer. Based on EWG's evaluation and the studies that support their stance, it would be good to take care with this ingredient.

Dr. Philippa Darbre's January 2012 study of 40 women showed that 99% of women's breast cancer tissues had one type of paraben in them.[305] This is why it became so important to find out if parabens have any association with breast cancer. Research by the EWG suggests that parabens are linked to organ toxicity, reproductive and fertility problems, birth and developmental defects, and hormone disruption. In 1998, 2004, and 2011, parabens were shown to mimic estrogen. [306] [307] [308] In 2001, they were shown to accelerate the growth of breast cancer cells[309] and in 2014 were proven to impair fertility.[310]

---

[305] Barr L, Darbre, PD et al. Mar 2012 *Journal of Applied Toxicology* "Measurement of paraben concentrations in human breast tissue at serial locations across the breast from axilla to sternum."

[306] Routledge EJ, et al Nov 1998 *Toxicol Appl Pharmacol* "Some alkyl hydroxyl benzoate preservatives (parabens) are estrogenic."

[307] Harvey PW and Everett DJ Jan 2004. *Journal of Applied Toxicology* "Significance

Ongoing studies show that parabens can enable hallmarks and characteristics of cancer in the human breast. Recent studies in 2014 demonstrate that parabens can activate four of the six hallmarks of breast cancer. These include causing DNA damage at high concentrations, genetic alterations and long term exposure to invasive activity in breast cancer cells.[311][312] A study in 2015 by Wrobel AM shows the actual pathways parabens use to alter breast cancer cells![313] Even though there are enough studies to show parabens are estrogenic and they can affect breast cancer cells, there are not enough studies on animals and humans, so no regulation has occurred at this point. The FDA labels parabens as Generally Recognized as Safe (GRAS). This is why this chemical can be found in your food as well as other products.

Since other ingredients that mimic estrogen are typically combined with parabens in our cosmetics, food and body products, we can easily eliminate parabens as well. Not only should it be eliminated from your food source, but also from being in contact with your skin. Dr. Joseph

of the detection of esters of p-hydroxybenzoic acid (parabens) in human breast tumors".

[308] Kim TS, Kim CY et al. Sep 2011 *Toxicol Res* "Estrogenic Activity of Persistent Organic Pollutants and Parabens Based on the Stably Transfected Human Estrogen Receptor-a Transcriptional Activation Assay (OECD TG 455)."

[309] Okubo T et al. Dec 2001 *Food Chem Toxicol* "ER-dependent estrogenic activity of parabens assessed by proliferation of human breast cancer MCF-7 cells and expression of ERalpha and PR."

[310] Braun JN, Just AC et al. Sep 2014 *J Expo Sci Environ Epidemiol* "Personal care product use and urinary phthalate metabolite and paraben concentrations during pregnancy among women from a fertility clinic."

[311] Darbre PD and Harvey PW Sep 2014 *J Appl Toxicol* "Parabens can enable hallmarks and characteristics of cancer in human breast epithelial cells: a review of the literature with reference to new exposure data and regulatory status."

[312] Wrobel AM and Gregoraszczuk E Nov 2014 *Toxicol Lett* "Actions of methyl-, propyl- and butylparaben on estrogen receptor-a and –b and the progesterone receptor in MCF-7 cancer cells and non-cancerous MCF-10A cells."

[313] Wrobel A and Gregoraszczuk E Aug 2015 *Toxicol Lett* "Action of methyl-, propyl- and butylparaben on GPR30 gene and protein expression, cAMP levels and activation of ERK1/2 and PI3KAkt signaling pathways in MC-7 breast cancer cells and MCF-10A non-transformed breast epithelial cells."

Mercola points out seven ingredients to avoid at http://bathcare.mercola.com/, one of which is paraben. Parabens are yet another reason to evaluate and change all lotions, soaps, hair products and deodorant to products sans chemicals. I was happy to find that parabens are bio-degradable, do not show up in our drinking water and will lower immediately upon lowering input in the body.[314]

I started re-evaluating the more frequently used products we put on our body, like lotions, deodorant, shampoo, conditioner and soap. Then I evaluated cosmetics. Lipstick was first, since it is estimated that we eat a significant amount of lipstick per year. Next was face lotion and cover up.

I sampled a number of facial skin products and *Origins* was a favorite. *Origins* products are rated about a four (the lower the better) by the EWG because some of the ingredients in them may have allergenic affects. I also use *Bausc's* skin care products. My favorites from *Bausc* are the under eye cream, lotion, body wash, deodorant, and children's products, all absolutely paraben, phthalate, gluten and chemical free. One of my clients told me about *SanRe*. It appears to have good skincare products and rates from 0 to 2 on the EWG website. I have not personally tried them, so I can't tell you if they work well or have pleasant odors.

Yes to Cucumbers and *Shea Moisture* shampoo and conditioner work great for hair and smell good. Dyeing your hair can also have toxic effects from the absorption and inhalation of chemicals, however, hair dye is not used on an everyday basis. Also, there are natural hair dye products that may help reduce this intake. Even though I chose to still dye my hair, I was still able to get rid of my breast lump.

My next changes are shadow, mascara and blush. I use those sparingly so I haven't changed those yet! I don't wear perfume or hair spray and I

---

[314] Haman C et al. Jan 2015 *Water Res* "Occurrence, fate and behavior of parabens in aquatic environments: a review."

rarely put on nail polish so I am not too worried about those, but they do have phthalate free nail polish products available.

You can look up any skincare, hair or oral care chemicals on www.ewg.org to find out their toxicity rating. Typically, you would want to use a product that has a rating of four or below.

Eradicate 4: PERFLUORINATED COMPOUNDS (PFCs)

PFCs are grease resistant coatings used in cookware, shampoos, floor wax, food wrapping, carpet treatments and other products. PFCs are commonly used on Teflon pans. They are also present in the air and water as industrial waste from chemical plants. PFCs can be ingested, inhaled and absorbed through the skin.

95% of Americans have PFOA, a type of PFC compound, in their blood. [315] PFCs have a long history of health problems. They have been linked to lower birth weight, abnormal thyroid levels, infertility, kidney and prostate cancer and tumor growth. Unlike other estrogenic chemicals that bind to fats, PFCs bind to blood proteins and therefore accumulate in the liver, kidneys and bile.

A March 2014 study on Greenlandic Inuit women studied genes involved in estrogen synthesis and xenobiotic metabolism. They discovered that two genes associated with breast cancer risk, when found with increased levels of perfluorooctane sulfonate (PFOS) and perfluorooctanoic acid (PFOA), caused an increased breast cancer risk. [316] PFOS are *Scotchguard* type of materials and PFOA is the chemical used in Teflon pans, carpet cleaning solutions, stain resistant carpets and microwave popcorn bags.

---

[315] Dr. Joseph Mercola Feb 2009 www.mercola.com "Common Chemicals Linked to Infertility".

[316] Ghisari M et al. Mar 2014 *Environ Health* "Polymorphisms in phase I and phase II genes and breast cancer risk and relations to persistent organic pollutant exposure: a case-control study in Inuit women."

Not only did PFCs increase risk in humans that have breast cancer genes, PFCs changed mammary gland growth, differentiation of terminal end buds, ductal branching as well as tumor incidence following treatment. A recent study in 2015 showed that PFOS and PFOA enhance the estrogenic effects of estradiol in human breast cancer cells.[317]

In May 2000, 3M announced they were phasing out PFOA, PFOS and PFOS-related products. Due to this, in 2002, DuPont built its own plant in NC to manufacture the chemical. A settlement of $235 million was awarded to those who brought action against DuPont in the area due to contamination of drinking water and related cancers. The EPA has since designated PFCs as a likely human carcinogen and set the advisory level of PFCs at 0.4 parts per billion in drinking water.

It may be difficult to get rid of PFCs entirely because they are resistant to biodegradation and stay in the environment for a while, but, there are things you can eliminate out of your home. Non-stick cookware such as Teflon pans, microwave popcorn bags, packaging for greasy foods, carpet and fabric protectors and flame retardants can all be removed. More and more we are seeing companies produce carpeting and furniture without PFCs and other chemicals in them. These ingredients may not always be listed but you can find products that advertise as *PFOA free*. A way to work around getting rid of furniture that has PFCs in them, is to cover them with fabric covers without PFCs.

Ceramic and glass pans are good alternatives for cooking. Ceramic pans and baking dishes are becoming more popular and these are readily available. Filtering your water will get PFCs out, so you will want to read the filtering comparison at the end of this chapter.

Eradicate 5: METALLOESTROGENS

---

[317] Sonthithai P et al. Aug 2015 J Appl Toxicol "Perfluorinated chemicals, PFOS and PFOA, enhance the estrogenic effects of 17β-estradiol in T47D human breast cancer cells."

Once again, there is another new "gen" term that indicates our internal battle against hormones. It is *metalloestrogens*. Scientists have found that many metals can have estrogenic effects. They have been shown to activate estrogen receptors when estradiol is not present. Estradiol production goes down after menopause which is perhaps why these metals start taking its place.

Metalloestrogens include cadmium, calcium, cobalt, copper, nickel, chromium, lead, mercury and tin. We have the largest exposure to aluminum, mercury, cadmium, arsenic and copper, so these are the ones I reviewed in this section. These metals can be present in your water, food and house air, basically anywhere in the environment. Metal exposure has increased over the last 50 to 60 years and many of these metals have a long biological life (cadmium has a half-life of 10 to 30 years).

Not only do they have a long life, but they can accumulate in the body and breast tissue.[318] In a 2003 study, copper, cobalt, nickel, lead, mercury, tin and chromium all had the ability to alter gene expression and increase estradiol.[319] Not only do they individually cause disruption to the hormone system, but there is evidence that these metals may work together to attack various cell processes, all working to create and grow breast cancer. Testing is available for these metals, if you decide to look into this further. I also had metal testing done and was high in mercury.

---

[318] Mohammadi M et al. 2014 *J Toxicol* "Concentration of cd, pb, hg, and se in different parts of human breast cancer tissues".
[319] Martin MB et al. Jun 2003 *Endocrinology* "Estrogen-like activity of metals in CF-7 breast cancer cells".

Aluminum

Aluminum is a concern because our exposure is highest to this metal. Aluminum can be found in drinking water, wine, food additives, cooking pans, drinking bottles, antacids, vaccines and deodorant. Aluminum has been measured in the human breast at levels higher than in blood.[320] These levels may be high enough to influence breast cells, including estrogen actions.

In 2008, the National Cancer Institute said that the results of studies were conflicting and there is not enough evidence to support aluminum or antiperspirants causing breast cancer. Many previous studies focused solely on aluminum in antiperspirants.[321] This is only a very small source of aluminum exposure throughout our lives, so I believe more studies are needed that include other sources.

Since the National Cancer Institute's statement in 2008, scientists have found that aluminum does indeed change the hormonal system. In 2010, a study on female fish demonstrated that aluminum can be an endocrine disruptor. [322] Additionally, in 2012 a study demonstrated that long term aluminum exposure caused increased estrogen, follicle stimulating hormone (FSH) and luteinizing hormone (LH) in the blood of female rats. These increases affected reproductive function in rats. [323] In 2013, studies by Darbre, PD showed that high amounts of aluminum were found in breast tissue and that aluminum can increase invasive properties of breast cancer cells. [324]

---

[320] Darbre PD, Mannello F and Exley C Nov 2013 *J Inor Biochem* "Aluminum and breast cancer: Sources of exposure, tissue measurements and mechanisms of toxicological actions on breast biology."

[321] Darbre PD Sep 2005 *J Inorg Biochem* "Aluminum, antiperspirants and breast cancer."

[322] Correia TG et al. May 2010 *Comp Biochem Physio CToxicol Pharmacol* "Aluminum as an endocrine disruptor in female Nile tilapia (Oreochromis niloticus)."

[323] Wang N et al. Mar 2012 *Biol Trace Elem Res.* "Effects of subchronic aluminum exposure on the reproductive function in female rats."

[324] Darbre PD, Bakir A and Iskakova E Nov 2013 *J Inorg Biochem* "Effect of aluminum on migratory and invasive properties of MCF-7 human breast cancer cells in

Aluminum can accumulate in the body, particularly the bone. Most recently, it is becoming clearer why aluminum may play a role in breast cancer. There is evidence that indicates aluminum displaces iron from its protein which raises the levels of free iron in the breast. [325] Breast cancer patients are known to have free iron levels five times higher than women without breast cancer. Free iron can trigger severe inflammation and free radicals, which can induce malignant tumor formation over time.

Still, more research needs to be done on cells to determine if breast cancer tissue is affected by the aluminum levels found in normal tissue. Even though there is not enough evidence to show aluminum directly effects or causes breast cancer in humans, we do know that aluminum can increase estrogen, along with other hormones, increases free iron, change properties of breast cancer cells and cause genetic changes. This is sufficient enough evidence to take a cautious approach to this metal.

When we are young, a significant source is from vaccines. Vaccines are imperative for the health of our society from major diseases, but some vaccines may not be as critical. This is why looking into each vaccine is so important to keep aluminum exposure down.

Ingested aluminum is another source of exposure. A main source of aluminum is alcoholic drinks. You've already seen how alcohol affects breast cancer, so it is important to keep alcohol intake low. We can get rid of aluminum pans and drinking bottles to decrease intake. Even stainless steel cookware can leach metals like aluminum and nickel. Stainless steel alloys all contain nickel, chromium, molybdenum, iron, carbon, and various other metals. In addition, higher temperatures will always increase the rate of leaching. One way you can tell if your pans have high levels of nickel in them is if they are not magnetized. If a

culture."
[325] Dr. Joseph Mercola Mar 2011 www.mercola.com "NEW Studies Reveal Alarming Hidden Cause of Breast Cancer".

magnet sticks to your pan, nickel content is low. Pans made of zirconium are considered a safe alternative.

Skin products contain high levels of aluminum, including deodorants. It took me a while to find good quality chemical and metal free skincare products. Many of them just smell bad or don't moisturize that well. Deodorant was the most difficult. I found two interesting facts about natural deodorants. One is that baking soda works well to keep odors away, but not moisture. If you sweat a lot, eventually the baking soda will not work anymore. You need to keep re-applying it all day long if you are going to use it by itself. Be aware that some baking powders have aluminum in them as an additive, so check labels!

The other interesting fact is that salt keeps you from sweating. Sodium chloride and sodium stearate both are rated 0 and 1, respectively, for toxicity on the EWG website and do the job of keeping perspiration at bay for most of the day. What I did at first was use two deodorants; one with salt and the other with baking soda. I used *Herban Cowboy's* unscented maximum protection deodorant (sodium stearate) along with *Bausc's* line of deodorant that has baking soda in it. *Bausc's* product is a soft powder and smells like mint and cucumbers. Other products that I use now and seem to work well for most of the day are *Desert Essence* tea tree oil deodorant, *Jason's* deodorant stick with sodium stearate, zinc and lavender and *Naturally Fresh* roll-on. I still need to re-apply these later in the day if it is hot outside but overall, I am happy with the way they work.

Arsenic

Arsenic is a metal primarily used along with other metals to stabilize them. A compound of arsenic is used in the production of pesticides, herbicides, insecticides and treated wood products. Even though the use of lead-arsenate insecticide was banned in the 1980s, residues are still found in the soil. MSMA, another arsenical pesticide, is still being used on golf courses, sod farms and highway right-of-ways. Further still, arsenical ingredients are permitted and found in animal feed to prevent diseases. Because of these uses, arsenic is found as a contaminant in groundwater and some meat, vegetables and fruit.

Research in 2007 found that 137 million people in more than 70 countries are most likely affected by arsenic poisoning of drinking water. [326] Contamination is found right here in the US. Our country set a new limit for arsenic in 2006 of .01 mg/L arsenic compared to the previous .50 mg/L. The state of New Jersey has lowered their limit to even below this standard at .005 mg/L for arsenic in drinking water. After a limit change in 2001, Arizona had approximately 35% of water supply wells out of compliance. California had 38%. Public water supply companies had to find alternative sources of water or better filtration systems.

Unfortunately, there is no set limit of arsenic in foods. *Consumer Reports* did a study in 2012 on more than 200 rice products and found high amounts of arsenic in many of them, including organic, Trader Joes and Whole Foods.[327] This was after their previous finding that arsenic was in apple and grape juices. Evidently, arsenic sticks to the shell of brown rice more so than white rice, so brown rice arsenic values are higher. Rice grown in Arkansas, Louisiana, Missouri and Texas, which accounts for 76% of US grown rice, generally had higher levels than rice grown elsewhere. Rice absorbs arsenic from soil and water much more effectively than most plants and this is why it is found in high amounts in rice. The EPA estimated in 2009, that 24% of our dietary arsenic comes from vegetables, 18% from fruits and juices and 17% from rice. The European Food Safety Authority found that rice cereal products account for half of our dietary exposure to inorganic arsenic.

A review by two scientists (Richard Stahlhut, MPH and Ana Navas-Acien, D, PhD) working with *Consumer Reports* found that of 3,633 participants, those eating one rice product per day had 44% higher urine or blood levels of arsenic. Those eating two or more rice products

---

[326] Aug 30 2007 www.USAToday.com "Arsenic in drinking water seen as threat"
[327] Nov 2012 www.consumerreports.org "Arsenic in Your Food".

per day had levels 70% higher. Because of these studies, Consumers Union, an advocacy arm of *Consumer Reports* and others are advocating the FDA to set limits in rice and juice products and even wine. The FDA has postponed any decisions until further research has been performed.

This is not to say that research on arsenic and breast cancer has not been performed. In a study on breast cancer cells in 2013, arsenic was the most toxic of four metals, with mercury following in second. [328] Arsenic is on EWG's top twelve list of endocrine disruptors. Arsenic is proven to be an endocrine disruptor in many cellular and animal studies and more are showing a link to breast cancer. A study in 2014 showed that breast cancer cells exposed to arsenic for six months had basal-like breast cancer characteristics, including ER and HER-2 and overexpression of two genes, p63 and K5. This study also showed an increase in estrogen and aromatase enzyme.[329] Aromatase enzyme is what controls the growth rate of estrogen.

Additionally, two recent population studies linked exposure to inorganic arsenic to breast cancer incidence. In Oct 2014, 2000 women in Mexico were tested for arsenic in their urine. This study showed that women who had high urinary levels of arsenic (believed to be from the drinking water) had an increased breast cancer risk.[330] The California Teachers Study, a large participant study consisting of 112,379 participants, reported in May 2015 that inorganic arsenic from ambient air may be a risk factor for breast cancer.[331] Who knows how many studies will need to be performed before arsenic is proven to be a contaminant in food, water and air, but based on these and many other

[328] Egiebor E et al. Oct 2013 *Int J Environ Res Public Health* "The kinetic signature of toxicity of four heavy metals and their mixtures on MCF7 breast cancer cell line".

[329] Xu Y et al. Feb 2014 *Arch Toxicol* "Arsenic-induced cancer cell phenotype in human breast epithelia is estrogen receptor-independent but involves aromatase activation".

[330] Lopez-Carrillo L et al. Oct 2014 *Toxicol Appl Pharmacol* "Arsenic methylation capacity is associated with breast cancer in northern Mexico."

[331] Liu R et al. May 2015 *Epidemiology* "Residential exposure to estrogen disrupting hazardous air pollutants and breast cancer risk: The California Teachers Study".

studies, it is safe to say that this metal should be avoided as much as possible as part of breast cancer prevention.

What can we do about arsenic in food? For now, we can research manufacturers to see what they are doing about it and where they are sourcing their rice. Some brands started testing their products after the *Consumer Reports* study was conducted. One of these is *Natures One*, a baby food manufacturer. They have managed to get most arsenic out of their products to nearly undetectable levels. Believe it or not, *Kellogg's Rice Krispies* tested lowest in the cereal category by *Consumer Reports* at 2.3 to 2.7 micrograms per serving. You can check out the study results at www.consumerreports.org or go to www.ewg.org to find products and shopping guides. Hopefully, I will have some of these products available on my web site soon so we can have one stop shopping for proestro free products (www.proestrofree.com).

We can also reduce our exposure to this metal in our food if we rinse rice, vegetables, fruit and potatoes prior to cooking and/or choose white rice, limit rice intake to one time per week, or try alternative grains such as quinoa, millet and amaranth. For arsenic in water, we can buy a good filter (see end of this section for more information). If you don't feel like buying a filter, you can test your water. Find a certified lab at Safe Drinking Water Hotline at 800-426-4791.

Lastly, some of you may be aware of arsenic in pressure treated wood. There are a few ways we can avoid ingesting arsenic from pressure treated wood around the house. You can seal decks and playground equipment built prior to February 2002 and wash hands after touching wood decks or equipment. Arsenic runs to the ground underneath the deck, so don't let your kids play in the soil there and if you are gardening, wear gloves. Never cut or sand this kind of wood and do not burn it in a fire.

Cadmium

Cadmium is a byproduct of zinc production found in industrial workplaces. Build-up of cadmium is mostly found in water, air and soil derived from zinc industries and their surroundings. It is released into the air from mining, battery manufacturing, metal soldering, welding, burning coal and household waste. In addition, 100mg/kg, which can lead to increased amounts in the soil. Among various sources of cadmium, the primary source in the environment is due to industrial contamination, which is mostly due to a byproduct of smelting. Smelting is the use of heat and chemicals to extract base metals from mined rocks. Because cadmium is being released into the air, cadmium in water and soil are increasing.

Cadmium is also found in small amounts in cigarettes. Studies show that people who smoke generally have twice the amount of cadmium than those who do not. There have been several recalls where cadmium has been found in drinking glasses sold by McDonald's and jewelry sold by Wal-Mart.

There is actually a disease called *itai-itai* in Japan. The cause of this disease was first documented in 1912 when people ingested rice containing cadmium due to contaminated irrigation water. The overdose of cadmium caused weak and brittle bones and spine and leg pain. In the US, cadmium has been detected at about 70% at hazardous waste sites. A survey revealed that 100% of surface and ground water samples had high concentrations of cadmium in New Jersey. California, Colorado, Idaho and Maine also had high concentrations of cadmium in surface and ground water samples.

Although surface water may have high concentrations of cadmium, most drinking water does not, due to water treatment and processing. However, there is reason for concern because surface water goes directly on our food. Fluids only account for approximately 3.2% of our dietary intake of cadmium, but potatoes, grain and cereal account for up to 36% of our intake. In the US, cadmium exposure from diet is estimated from .12 to .331 ug/kgbw/day with the highest exposure to children one to six years old.

Compared to other countries, we may not be subjected to high levels of cadmium, but it does exist in our food at low levels everywhere. If you are living or have lived near an industrial plant, you will be subjected to higher levels of cadmium. 512,000 industry workers may be exposed to this metal. There are federal and state regulations in place for worker exposure as well as for air from waste sites. Even though there are regulations, the rules haven't always been as stringent. Since cadmium has a life of 10 to 30 years, cadmium is being re-circulated from air to soil to water. Its long life also explains why significant accumulation can happen in the body with low exposure over time.

There is no known use for cadmium in higher biological organisms. Cadmium is listed on the *European Restriction of Hazardous Substances*. The EPA has classified cadmium as group B-1, probable human carcinogen. Cadmium is known to cause effects on the lungs when inhaled in high amounts. Animal studies have linked cadmium exposure to lung, kidney, liver, bone, immune system, blood and nervous system effects. There are no federal limits to cadmium in food in the US to date.

Cadmium is the most studied of all the metalloestrogens. Occupational exposure has been linked to breast cancer by as much as 138% relative risk. Other studies have been performed on non-occupationally exposed women (dietary exposure), where scientists measure cadmium in urine. Those women with the highest levels of cadmium had a two-fold increased risk of breast cancer. A couple of these population studies performed in Long Island, New York and Wisconsin, actually estimated that 35% to 36% of breast cancer may be attributed to cadmium.[332] A 2012 population-based study showed that long term dietary intake of cadmium is associated with increased breast cancer

---

[332] Byrne C et al. Jan 2013 *J Mammary Gland Biol Neoplasia* "Metals and Breast Cancer".

risk in postmenopausal women.[333] This study was able to suggest the causal effect of cadmium in the development of breast cancer. Since this study, several other studies have shown a high risk of breast cancer with dietary intake of cadmium.[334] A Japanese study in 2013 showed an increase of 505% (odds ratio).[335] Others studies are linking cadmium directly to ER-positive and HER2 negative breast cancer.[336]

In addition to population studies, scientists reviewed scientific evidence for cadmium's estrogenic effects in 2012 and found that the cellular evidence was persuasive. [337] It is known to harm DNA directly and change the DNA repair system that helps repair cancer. Several studies show cadmium's estrogen growth effect on breast cancer cells and its increased expression on estrogen regulated genes. Causal effect of cadmium to breast cancer still needs additional research, but there is enough evidence to show that cadmium can activate estrogen receptors and that breast cancer and cadmium exposure are linked.

Our primary source of exposure is from industrial plants, cigarettes and food intake. We can avoid cadmium if we choose not to live near industrial plants, not smoke cigarettes, eat organic food grown in areas not near industrial plants and rinse our food with filtered water. Even if we live near industrial plants or waste sites, we can filter the water and choose to eat food not grown near home. Evidently, taking iron can negate the effects of cadmium. There are at least five studies that show iron decreases the absorption of cadmium in the stomach.[338] You can

---

[333] Julin B et al. Mar 2012 *Cancer Res* "Dietary cadmium exposure and risk of postmenopausal breast cancer: a population-based prospective cohort study".

[334] Itoh H et al. Jan 2014 *Int J Hyg Environ Health* "Dietary cadmium intake and breast cancer risk in Japanese women: a case-control study".

[335] Nagata C et al. Feb 2013 *Breast Cancer Res Treat* "Cadmium exposure and the risk of breast cancer in Japanese women".

[336] Strumylaite L et al. May 2014 *Breast Cancer Res Treat* "Association between cadmium and breast cancer risk according to estrogen receptor and human epidermal growth factor receptor 2: epidemiological evidence".

[337] Silva N, et al. May 2012 *J Appl Toxicol* "Cadmium a metalloestrogens: are we convinced?"

[338] Julin B, et al. 2011 *Environ Health* "Relation between dietary cadmium intake and

264

get a blood test to check ferritin (iron) levels to make sure they are adequate.

Copper

Copper is used in building materials, as a conductor of heat and electricity, and a metal alloy. It can also be found as a compound in fungicides, bacteriostatic substances and wood preservatives. We are exposed to copper primarily by drinking water from copper supply plumbing in the home. 98% of all homes built after 1970 have copper pipes.

Copper is the only metalloestrogen that is actually vital to our bodies. It is a key dietary mineral as it helps in the enzymatic process of respiration. At high levels, copper can be toxic and cause a host of symptoms including PMS, stomach pain, diarrhea, liver damage, fatigue, headaches, autism, childhood hyperactivity and depression.

In humans, copper is found in the liver, muscle and bone. Exposure to copper is typically from ingestion of water or vitamin supplements. If you have copper plumbing, some inorganic copper flakes go into your water.

Copper exposure has been linked to non-Hodgkin's lymphoma and skin cancer. Skin cancer happens to be a sister cancer to breast cancer, meaning that a high number of women with breast cancer also get skin cancer. We are seeing more and more that copper is related to breast cancer. At least eight studies show that higher concentrations of copper are found in the blood of breast cancer patients and that the highest amounts are found in advanced stages. Like other metals, copper, in studies, stimulated cell growth by utilizing estrogen receptors.[339] This may be good enough reason for women to avoid using the copper IUD,

biomarkers of cadmium exposure in premenopausal women accounting for the body iron stores".
[339] Martin MB et al. Jun 2003 *Endocrinology* "Estrogen-like activity of metals in MCF-7 breast cancer cells".

however, there have not been any studies to indicate that the copper in the IUD releases in large amounts into the blood stream. A helpful option is to get your metals tested with a urine test to determine if copper is an area of concern for you.

Amazingly, phase 1 and 2 human clinical trials utilizing a copper depletion drug, tetrathiomolybdate (known in the industry as TM), show how copper can affect the enzymatic pathways of cancer cells. These trials also show that depleting copper actually prevents relapse of triple-negative and stage 3 and 4 breast cancer. So far, clinical trials are demonstrating a survival rate of 85% by using this copper depleting drug.[340] [341] Normal survival rates for these types of patients have ranged from none to 75% over 5 years, depending on the type of cancer. Dr. Linda Vahdat, one of the study's senior investigators, believes that copper works by affecting the bone marrow-derived cells that are needed for tumor growth.[342] Instead of increasing the estrogen receptors as in estrogen receptor-positive breast cancer, copper takes the place of estradiol at the receptor sites! Here is another example that demonstrates proestros are causing breast cancer, maybe even triple negative.

On June 7, 1991, the EPA published a regulation to control lead and copper in drinking water. This regulation is known as the *Lead and Copper Rule*. The rule requires monitoring of drinking water at customers taps in their homes. If the copper concentration exceeds 1.3ppm in more than 10% of taps sampled, the water supply company would need to take additional action. Currently, the EPA is in an evaluation phase that should end by 2016 to determine if new limits are needed for copper and lead in water.

---

[340] Quinin Pan et al. Sep 2002 *Cancer Res* "Copper Deficiency Induced by Tetrathiomolybdate Suppresses Tumor Growth and Angiogenesis."

[341] Jain S et al. Jun 2013 *Ann Oncol* "Tetrathiomolybdate-associated copper depletion decreases circulating endothelial progenitor cells in women with breast cancer at high risk of relapse".

[342] Vahdat Linda et al. Feb 2013 *Weill Cornell Newsroom* "Copper Depletion Therapy Keeps High-Risk Triple-Negative Breast Cancer at Bay."

If you have a house with copper supply plumbing, all is not lost. You can limit your copper intake by installing a water filtration system designed to remove heavy metals. Another item we may not think of too much is copper cookware. If you are trying to limit copper intake, it would be a good idea to replace copper cookware with ceramic. Perhaps you could use the copper cookware as a decoration, garden container or trade it in at a recycle center for cash.

We may not think of supplements as containing copper, but many of them do. Make sure you are not taking a supplement that has copper in it, unless you are doing so under the supervision of a doctor. Many supplements use inorganic copper, which is a more toxic type.

Mercury

Half the mercury that exists in the atmosphere comes from natural sources such as volcanos. Another 40% is from combustion of coal. Mercury evaporates into the air then is absorbed into the oceans from these sources. Eventually it ends up in the fish that we eat. Mercury is used in thermometers, barometers, float valves, fluorescent lamps and other devices. Due to concerns about mercury's toxicity, it has been largely phased out of thermometers. It remains in use for some research applications, fluorescent bulbs, antiseptics, laxatives and metal dental fillings. Due to the European Union calling for compact fluorescent bulbs to be mandatory by 2012, China had to re-open a mine to obtain the mercury required for bulb manufacturing. Mercury was recently removed from most vaccines (known as *Thimerosal*), but it is still present in the influenza vaccine.

Mercury poisoning can occur due to inhalation of the vapor, direct contact or from eating seafood contaminated with mercury. Mercury is known to cause a whole host of problems including tremors, impaired thinking, sleep disturbance, chest pain and cough, but in regards to hormones, it can bind directly to a hormone that regulates the menstrual cycle and ovulation and interfere with normal hormonal pathways. Women who work in dentistry have increased frequency of fertility issues, breast cancer and reproductive organ cancer.[343]

Mercury is on EWG's top twelve list of endocrine disruptors. The EPA lists mercury as a probable carcinogen. In 1996, an act was passed to phase mercury out of batteries. In 1990, the US Clean Air Act put mercury on a list of toxic pollutants that needs to be controlled as much as possible. In 2002, the US Senate passed legislation to phase out the sale of mercury filled thermometers. In 2011, the EPA announced new rules for coal-fired plants. Several other countries have banned mercury in manufacturing or dental amalgams. There has not been enough data for action to be taken for mercury in over-the-counter drugs or cosmetics.

Believe it or not, mercury is widely used in mascara. Minnesota was the first state to ban added mercury in cosmetics. A study on mercury exposure in skin care products showed higher concentration levels in urine of women in New York who used mercury containing products. [344] For this reason, I have changed to a mercury free mascara.

Exposure to mercury can be decreased by making good choices in regards to fish, as discussed in Chapter 14. Having mercury fillings replaced by a specialist, choosing LED light bulbs, reading labels on laxatives and over the counter products and lastly, choosing cosmetics carefully are all ways to reduce mercury exposure. I had metals tested by urine excretion and mercury was the highest level of them all. I have since had my dental fillings removed and have been working on reducing this metal, as well as others from my body. It is important to find a dentist who will be able to employ precautions during the removal of fillings so that you are not exposed while the fillings are being taken out.

---

[343] Simning A and van Wijngaarden E Jul 2007 *Occup Environ Med* "Literature review of cancer mortality and incidence among dentists".

[344] McKelvey W et al. 2010 *Environ Health Perspect* "Population-Based Inorganic Mercury Biomonitoring and the Identification of Skin Care Products as a Source of Exposure in New York City".

Lead

Lead can be found in homes built prior to 1978, usually in paint, which can be inhaled or ingested. Exterior paint can also flake off into the ground surrounding the home. There are also older lead pipes and lead solder on copper pipes still in existence in some older homes. Those with the highest exposure to lead are workers who are exposed in industries where there is use of lead in the making of other products. Lead based paint, leaded gasoline and lead batteries have been phased out, so most people do not have high exposure to this metal. Even though products have been discontinued, lead can still show up in toxic waste dumps with demolition of buildings and then to the environment. Lead is monitored in public water systems via the "Lead and Copper Rule" by the EPA. The action level is .015.

Children are more susceptible to lead absorption than adults. Lead has been linked to nervous system, kidney and blood disorders, and to hormone disruption, and even breast cancer.[345] It is on EWG's top twelve list of endocrine disruptors due to the fact that in animals, it has been found to lower sex hormone levels and to disrupt the hormone signaling that regulates the major stress system. In 2010 a study found that higher levels of lead were found in blood and head hair samples of newly diagnosed breast cancer patients with infiltrating ductal carcinoma. They also found that lead and other metals interact with iodine, which most likely protects against breast cancer.[346] However, in a 2013 study where scientists compared four metals in breast cancer cells, lead was the least toxic. [347]

---

[345] Martin MB et al. June 2003 *Endocrinology* "Estrogen-like activity of metals in MCF-7 breast cancer cells".

[346] Alatise OI and Schrauzer GN 2010 *Biological Trace Element Research* "Lead exposure: A contributing cause of the current breast cancer epidemic in Nigerian Women".

[347] Egiebor E et al. Oct 2013 *Int J Environ Res Public Health* "The kinetic signature of toxicity of four heavy metals and their mixtures on MCG7 breast cancer cell line".

Because this metal is not as prevalent as others and it is fairly well contained, I won't go into much more detail on it. If you work in an industry using lead, have lead pipes or solder, make sure you are taking every precaution against inhalation or ingestion of this metal. If you are on public water, you can look up testing results to see how your community's water fared last year.

Eradicate 6: HOUSEHOLD CONTAMINENTS

Cleaning solvents can be another form of proestros in the home. Cleaning solvents such as dish soap, laundry detergent, furniture polish and surface cleaners can have harmful chemicals like phthalates, glycol esters, synthetic musks, styrene and formaldehyde and a host of other endocrine disrupting, cancer causing chemicals.

As seen previously with phthalates, human and animal research show many of the chemicals in cleaning products cause mammary-gland cancer and disrupt the endocrine system. Air fresheners are also on the list that contribute to proestros. A survey in 2010 found that women who used air fresheners and mold and mildew cleaners had double the risk of breast cancer. Approximately 1500 women were surveyed in Massachusetts. Half of the women had breast cancer and half did not. [348]

Nonylphenol ethoxylate (NPE) is a common ingredient in laundry detergent and all-purpose cleaners. This chemical is banned in Europe because it is known to be a potent endocrine disruptor. A study in 2004 showed that nonylphenols can bind to estrogen receptors in cells. [349]

These are just two of many harmful chemicals in cleaning products. If I researched each one, it would take me another few years to complete

---

[348] *The Columbus Dispatch* July 20, 2010 "Study suggests link of cleaners to breast cancer".

[349] Garcia-Revero N et al. Mar 2004 *Environ Toxicol Chem* "Estrogenic potential of halogenated derivatives of nonylphenol ethoxylates and carboxylates".

this book. It is best to use alternative products that are not potentially harmful to the body. The problem with trying to locate a safe alternative is that you won't know what is in the product based on reading labels. Manufacturers are not required to list their secret ingredients and many of them are toxic. The easy part of finding cleaners is to simply go back to basics. There are probably many items in your house right now that can be used. The ones I use are baking soda, vinegar and Borax. These are good for scrubbing bathtubs, toilets and sinks and are also better for septic systems.

For the kitchen, I make my own cleaner in a spray bottle. My recipe for cleaning counters is 2 tsp Borax, 2T Vinegar, 2C hot water, a few drops lemon oil, and a few drops lavender oil. Lavender oil is an anti-bacterial. I use lemon because I not a fan of the smell of lavender. Another cleaner Dr. Joseph Mercola recommends is hydrogen peroxide and vinegar mixed. You can put any of these into a spray bottle and there you have it! Vinegar can also be used as a natural fabric softener. Essential oils can be used as air freshener. Just make sure you are not getting fragrance oils. Those contain artificial ingredients.

Insecticides and herbicides are tools we use at home to get rid of those pesky bugs and weeds. As you know from the beginning of this book, organochlorines are the main ingredient in insecticides and herbicides, and are proestros. Generally, insecticides or herbicides are typically referred to collectively as pesticides. If you use these around your home and in your yard, you are exposing you, your neighbors and perhaps any people downstream from you to all these chemicals. I don't recommend using them, except in isolated containers.

A neighbor of mine did an experiment on stink bugs and found that a spray bottle with dish soap and water did just as well to kill the bugs than a leading insecticide. It works by suffocating them. Well there must be some potent stuff in that dish soap! We know that a lot of detergents have phthalates which are also endocrine disruptors.

Diatomaceous earth, a white powder, is a great natural alternative for lawn insects, fleas and ticks. You may have heard that it can also be taken internally and used as a natural detoxifier for the body. As an all-natural ingredient from the ocean, there are still precautions to take. A mask is recommended while spreading it because it is considered an irritant for the lungs. Diatomaceous earth works by eroding exoskeletons. It kills just as many bugs as the leading lawn insecticide and I have never found a flea one on my cats! In fact, you can put it on your pet's fur to keep fleas and ticks away.

Vodka in a spray bottle can kill wasps and bees. A Japanese beetle bag is about the only pesticide I use because it is contained inside a bag. There are other home remedies where bugs will be drawn to the insecticide inside an old soda or milk jug and then die inside the container. I have found these remedies for mosquitoes, drain flies and other flying insects.

As far as weeds, my battle goes as far as this: I eat dandelions with salads and over seed with grass seeds in the spring and the fall. I hand pull weeds in the garden bed and cover in with mulch or leftover bark from fallen trees. That seems to keep the weeds down enough. I add landscape cloth or newspaper over areas where I am going to mulch or lay stone to keep weeds down in those areas.

Flame Retardants

Flame retardants are used in electronics like cell phones, alarm clocks, and computers but are also found in foam in our couch cushions, carpet padding and mattresses. They can also be found on some textiles, such as curtains, and in appliances, such as refrigerators. Flame retardants are put in products to help prevent overheating and to make them less flammable. Back in the 70s, flame retardants were put in children's clothing...until they found out there were health issues associated with it. I used to have a night gown with a flame retardant label which was given to me by my grandparents!

The first version of flame retardant was PBDE (Decabrominated diphenyl ether), which is an organobromine compound. These are structurally like PCBs. Scientists have found this chemical in our bodies as well as wildlife worldwide. The amount has been doubling in our bodies every five years since 1972.

How does it get in our body in the first place? The primary route is through inhalation of dust particles that collect in the home. In our body, it accumulates in our blood, fat and breast milk and is resistant to degradation. Evidence has shown that PBDE is linked to decreased fertility, brain developmental problems, hyperthyroid and even cancer. A study in 2012 showed that PBDE was able to promote the growth of breast, ovarian and cervical cancer cells and even inhibit the effects of the drug *tamoxifen*.[350] Because evidence has shown PBDE stays in the environment and causes hormonal disruption, PBDE has virtually been eliminated from production. Two forms of this flame retardant have been banned from manufacture in the US.

The replacement and most heavily produced flame retardant in the world is TBBPA (Tetrabromobisphenol-A). Notice "bisphenol-A" within this term? This type of flame retardant actually degrades to BPA and dimethyl ether. TBBPA acts similarly to BPA as discussed previously. It has recently been found to be associated with hormonal cancer and disruption, although studies are mixed. According to the EWG, some studies have shown evidence that it may interfere with estrogens and androgens. EWG also pointed out a cellular study in 2013 that showed how TBBPA might cause uterine cancer.[351]

Las Pedersen of NIEHS Laboratory of Structural Biology states that TBBPA may raise levels of estradiol in the body due to its ability to compete with binding receptors. This is based on cellular studies in the

---

[350] Li ZH et al. Apr 2012 *Environ Health Perspect* "Effects of decabrominated diphenyl ether (BDE-209) in regulation of growth and apoptosis of breast, ovarian, and cervical cells".

[351] Gosavi RA et al. Oct 2013 *Environ Health Prospect* "Mimicking of Estradiol Binding by Flame Retardants and Their Metabolites: A Crystallographic Analysis".

lab.[352] It has not been tested on humans. Heather Stapleton, an associate professor of environmental chemistry at Duke and Butt's says "Having continuous exposure to man-made chemicals that can bind with the same affinity as endogenous hormones may have very significant consequences on development and overall health".

With the evidence we have available, it would be wise to reduce levels of flame retardants in our homes as much as possible. One of things we can do is dust often with a wet rag and vacuum with a HEPA filter. We can avoid reupholstering furniture on our own. We can try to buy products without flame retardants. We can choose products that are made with less flammable materials such as down, wool, and cotton. We can wear a mask when working with insulation or entering attics. We can wash our hands after handling electrical equipment such as TVs, laptops, toner cartridges and cell phones. Lastly, we can look for "green" building materials when buying new carpeting, padding, mattresses and upholstery. Some products state they are flame retardant free.

Eradicate 7: EXTERIOR POLLUTANTS

PAHs (polycyclic aromatic hydrocarbons) are a group of 200 chemicals that are formed when coal, wood, gasoline, oil, garbage, fat, incense or tobacco is burned. In nature, PAHs can be found in coal, crude oil and from forest fires and volcanoes. PAH can also be found in food when meats are cooked over a high flame. PAHs are less water-soluble and mix more easily with oily substances. They can be found in the air as they attach to sediment in the air. PAH is found at increasing levels worldwide due to our increasing use of natural fuels and vehicles, combined with its natural existence. However, unlike some other external proestros, PAH is broken down in the environment by reacting with sunlight and other chemicals over a few days to weeks. Bacteria can break it down in the soil and water over a few weeks to months.

---

[352] Kelly S. Betts Oct 2013 *Science Selections* "Molecular Competition Flame Retardants Interact with Key Metabolism Enzyme".

There are still other PAHs that can take years to break down in soil and ground water.

In a 2003 Silent Spring Institute study, three types of PAHS were found in more than three-quarters of homes dust samples.[353] Inhalation is the primary route of exposure to the body. Seven types of PAH have been identified by the EPA as probable human carcinogens. One type of PAH called benzopyrene has been widely studied because it's the main by-product in cigarette smoke. According to the EPA website, population studies have reported an increase in lung cancer in humans exposed to coal coke oven emissions, roofing tar emissions and cigarette smoke.

PAH's link with lung cancer is clear. The link to breast cancer however is not without conflict. Since PAHs are fat seeking, they can be stored in the fat tissue of the breast. The most common PAHs (benzanthracene and benzopyrene) were shown in 2005 to be mildly estrogenic by way of interacting with the estrogen receptor.[354] Some PAHs are known to actually cause DNA mutations and a recent cellular study in May 2015, even showed what signals benzopyrene may be using to form human breast cancer cells.[355]

More and more studies are linking PAH exposure to breast cancer. Scientists in 1999 showed a correlation between workplace-exposed individuals and pre-menopausal breast cancer.[356] An important recent population study found that exposure to PAHs was associated with

[353] Rudel RA et al. Oct 2003 *Environ Sci Technology* "Phthalates, alkylphenols, pesticides, polybrominated diphenyl ethers, and other endocrine-disrupting compounds in indoor air and dust".

[354] Pliskova M et al. Feb 2005 *Toxicol Science* "Deregulation of cell proliferation by polycyclic aromatic hydrocarbons in human breast carcinoma MCF-7 cells reflects both genotoxic and nongenotoxic events".

[355] Guo J et al. May 2015 *Toxicol Lett* "Effects of exposure to benzopyrene on metastasis of breast cancer are mediated through ROS-ERK-MMP9 axis signaling".

[356] Petrallia SA et al. Jun 1999 *Scan J Work Environ Health* "Risk of premenopausal breast cancer in association with occupational exposure to polycyclic aromatic hydrocarbons and benzene".

mutations of the p53 tumor suppressor gene in breast cancer cellular samples.[357]

Several studies have demonstrated that PAH caused breast tumors in lab animals. Two reports showed correlations between human death from breast cancer and PAH exposure. One in Taiwan in 2012 showed that those living in areas with high PAH particulate in the air had an increased probability of dying from breast cancer.[358] The second report from the Long Island Study in 2009 showed that those breast cancer patients who had high levels of PAH-DNA in their ducts and had also received radiation, had an increased risk of death.[359] Those taking hormone therapy as part of their treatment had an increased survival rate. Another review in 2015 from the Long Island Study linked vehicular traffic-related exposure to breast cancer incidence.[360] Suffice to say, there is sufficient evidence to indicate PAH as a proestro.

Federal vehicle emission standards have led to a decrease of PAH release by vehicles compared to their highest levels in the 1970s according to a study by Beyea in 2008.[361] OSHA regulates PAH exposure in the workplace. NIOSH (National Institute for Occupational Safety and Health) monitors other work sites such as asphalt paving. The EPA requires that industries report environmental releases of PAH that are more than one pound. For instance, the EPA monitored PAH released from the Gulf oil spill.

It seems that we have plenty of regulatory bodies monitoring PAHs in our environment, but there are still things we can do ourselves to lower

[357] www.breastcancerfund.org "Polycyclic Aromatic Hydrocarbons (PAHs)"

[358] Hung Li-Ju et al. 2012 *Aerosol and Air Quality Research* "Traffic Air Pollution and Risk of Death from Breast Cancer in Taiwan: Fine particulate Matter (PM2.5) as a Proxy Marker".

[359] Sagiv SK et al. Apr 2009 *Environ Res* "Polycyclic aromatic hydrocarbon-DA adducts and survival among women with breast cancer".

[360] Modukhovich I et al. May 2015 *Environ Health Perspect* "Vehicular Traffic-Related Polycyclic Aromatic Hydrocarbon Exposure and Breast Cancer Incidence: The Long Island Breast Cancer Study Project (LIBCSP)".

[361] www.breastcancerfund.org "Polycyclic Aromatic Hydrocarbons (PAHs)

our exposure around us. We can avoid breathing in car exhaust by turning on the air recirculate button and closing car windows if there are trucks or smoking cars nearby. This will keep the smoke out of the vehicle. We can avoid being near a stand-alone propane or kerosene heater, camp fire or wood stove and make sure combustible appliances are well vented to the outside air.[362] We can choose not to use synthetic wood logs for burning. We can avoid burning garbage, especially tires. We can choose to not burn incense or smoke.

We can avoid eating meat that has been overcooked. We can cook meats on low on the grill. We can avoid getting tattoos because the black ink has tar in it. We can avoid body lotions or anti-dandruff shampoo with tar in them. We can use personal protective equipment while sealing an asphalt driveway, or cleaning a chimney or asphalting a roof. Lastly, we can properly dispose of oil, gas, diesel fuel and creosote to prevent soil and water contamination.

Smoking: Thankfully, smoking has been on the decline as one of our major external proestro contributors since the 1960s. Only about 12% of adults smoke nowadays, where it used to be 43%. Not only are we exposed to the chemicals in cigarette smoke through smoking ourselves, but also through second hand smoke. There are at least 70 chemicals in cigarette smoke that are considered carcinogenic. A number of these chemicals have more recently been linked to breast cancer.[363]

Several studies indicate that women who begin smoking cigarettes within five years of starting their period or five years prior to their first pregnancy, have a much higher risk of breast cancer.[364] [365]Two large

---

[362] White AJ et al. Dec 2014 *Environ Health* "Indoor air pollution exposure from use of indoor stoves and fireplaces in association with breast cancer: a case-control study".

[363] www.breastcancerfund.org "Tobacco Smoke: Active and Passive Exposures"

[364] Band PR et al. Oct 2002 *Lancet* "Carcinogenic and endocrine disrupting effects of cigarette smoke and risk of breast cancer".

[365] Catsburg C et al. May 2015 *Int J Cancer* "Active cigarette smoking and risk of breast cancer".

population studies, including the Nurses' Health Study[366] and Women's Health Initiative Study in 2011 which involved over 80,000 participants each, showed that breast cancer incidence is higher in those who smoke for a longer period of time and have increased number of cigarettes per day.[367] [368]

Another report in 2011, analyzed smoking and sex hormones and found that smoking was related to higher levels of estradiol, other steroid hormones and testosterone (which is a source of estrogen when metabolized).[369] A 2014 population study linked long-term, current and recent smokers to estrogen receptor-positive breast cancer in pre-menopausal women.[370]

As mentioned previously, benzopyrene, a PAH in smoke, is carcinogenic to cells that line milk ducts, is estrogenic and has been linked to breast cancer. In a 2013 study, benzopyrene at high concentrations affected the DNA that causes breast cancer growth in human cells.[371] Benzopyrenes are detected in urban air at twice the amount than rural air.

Acrylamide is another chemical found in cigarette smoke. It is also found in foods cooked at high temperatures, such as French fries. It is not yet clear if it causes breast cancer, but ingestion of acrylamide has been linked to breast cancer in cellular, animal and population studies. In human population studies, dietary exposure has been shown to be

---

[366] Colditz GA Mar 1995 J Am Med Womens Assoc "The nurses' health study: a cohort of US women followed since 1976".

[367] Xue F et al. Jan 2011 Arch Intern Med "Cigarette smoking and the incidence of breast cancer".

[368] Luo J et al. Mar 2011 BMJ "Association of active and passive smoking with risk of breast cancer among postmenopausal women: a prospective cohort study".

[369] Band PR et al. Oct 2002 Lancet "Carcinogenic and endocrine disrupting effects of cigarette smoke and risk of breast cancer".

[370] Kawai M et al. Apr 2014 Cancer "Active smoking and the risk of estrogen receptor-positive and triple-negative breast cancer among women ages 20 to 44 years".

[371] Chen Y et al. Feb 2013 Toxicology "Benzo[a]pyrene repressed DNA mismatch repair in human breast cancer cells".

related to endocrine related tumors such as estrogen positive breast cancer. Additionally, exposure to acrylamide was linked to death of estrogen positive Danish women with breast cancer by 123% in 2012.[372]

In addition to these two proestros (benzopyrene and acrylamide), cigarettes contain vinyl chloride which has already been discussed previously as an endocrine disruptor. The tobacco leaves in cigarettes also have radioactive particles according to www.cancer.org. These particles (polonium-210) become present in smoke and enter the lungs. Over time the particles build up in the lungs, which can mean a big dose of radiation.

Many studies that link breast cancer to smoking show an increased risk among those who started smoking at an early age and those who smoked more than 20 cigarettes per day for a long period of time. According to the Band, PR study in 2002, this may "suggest that cigarette smoke exerts a dual action on the breast, with different effects in premenopausal and postmenopausal women".[373]

The best thing to do is avoid cigarette smoke by not smoking and avoid sitting near someone who is smoking. The new vapor cigarettes have a fraction of the chemicals that regular tobacco smoke has and "are a safer alternative" says Michael Siegel, M.D., MPH, a professor at Boston University's School of Health. That doesn't mean we should all start "vaping" because they come with side effects from the nicotine itself, but they are safer.

Electromagnetic radiation

Light waves and other types of energy that radiate from where they're produced are called *electromagnetic radiation*. Together, they make up what's known as the electromagnetic spectrum. The electromagnetic

---

[372] Olsen A et al. Jun 2012 *Toxicology* "Pre-diagnostic acrylamide exposure and survival after breast cancer among postmenopausal Danish women".
[373] Band PR et al. Oct 2002 *Lancet* "Carcinogenic and endocrine disrupting effects of cigarette smoke and risk of breast cancer".

spectrum contains all the different forms of electric and magnetic energies that vibrate from side to side traveling in a straight direction at the speed of light. Well-known forms of energy include: radio waves (cell phone towers), microwaves, infrared, ultraviolet, x-rays, and gamma rays. Some of these energy forms are man-made and some are natural. Human cells actually emit energy waves similar to a wavelength of microwaves. Electromagnetic waves similar to microwaves hitting the body over long periods of time, can disrupt the body's own energy waves. What affects energy waves have on the body depend on the wavelength, the proximity to the body and the length of exposure.

High frequency x-rays and are well-studied and are a known cause of breast cancer. Common examples of high dose radiation (10 to 8000 rads) are medical chest x-rays used for scoliosis, tuberculosis and cancer treatment itself. Common low exposure x-rays are airline check through points, flights, smoking and mammograms.

Short wavelengths take longer to affect the body. These wavelengths are typically referred to as *electromagnetic frequencies* (EMF). Electromagnetic radiation, even short frequency, is historically known to cause biological consequences, even when meeting the existing US regulations. Over time, we are increasingly exposed to electromagnetic frequencies (EMF) due to advances in technology and increasing use of wireless devices. Electromagnetic pollution from electric and magnetic energy is produced mostly by electronics and transmitters and can sometimes be caused by old power line's failure to conduct electricity back to transformers.

The history of electromagnetic radiation and its effects on the human body have been well documented in more recent years. In 1990, non-industry funded studies linked cancer to power lines. In 1992, the IEEE standard for electromagnetic frequencies was developed for commercial buildings. In 2003, non-industry funded studies linked cell phones to brain cancer.

Even though studies have shown EMF can cause illness in humans, levels are increasing more each year. In 2008, fluorescent lights were found to emit high electromagnetic frequencies. As of July 2014, 50 million "smart meters" have been installed on the outside of houses nationwide, which utilize wireless technology to transmit data from your appliances and to other smart meters. This is equivalent to 43% of the US. There is an option to opt out of installation of a smart meter, but you may have to pay a monthly fee.

With the increase in wireless technology, people are starting to have electromagnetic hypersensitivity (electro sensitivity) from all the technology emitting these magnetic and radio frequencies. Those products that can affect us daily are wireless phones, Wi-Fi, battery chargers, fluorescent light bulbs, smart meters, wireless transmitter tower, kitchen appliances, televisions, computers and clock radios. Even though electromagnetic fields rapidly decrease with distance, many of these items are used close to the body and for long periods of time. Even though studies have been conflicting, a report by the California Health Department concluded that electromagnetic fields are likely to cause adult leukemia, brain cancers and possibly breast cancer and could be responsible for one tenth of all miscarriages.[374]

Cell phones, in particular are becoming newsworthy due to their proximity to the body and link to cancers. Cell phones have a significant amount of electromagnetic frequencies surrounding them. Doctors like Dr. John West, who appeared on the Dr. Oz Show, are finding breast tumors shaped like cell phones in more and more woman at young ages who wear their cell phone under their bra! These women got breast cancer at age 21 from wearing their cell phone in their bra for ten hours per day. Cell phones have specific instructions to not be held close to the body (iPhone 5 is 3/8"). You do not want to leave a cell phone near your head at night or tuck a cell phone in your bra or pocket for any length of time! There's a reason why we get a weird ringing feeling in

[374] Havas Magda 2004 *Electromagnetic Environments and Health in Buildings* Chapter 10 "Biological Effects of Low Frequency Electromagnetic Fields".

our leg or side when we wear your phone next to your body regularly. Another way to avoid cell phone radiation is to use a hands free option like speaker phone, blue-tooth or headphones.

Many of us use computers on a daily basis. Laptops sold today have wireless transmitters and antennas that emit radiofrequency radiation (also known as wireless radiation) to transfer data. The computer is configured to use this wireless technology whether you operate a wireless or cabled computer network.

When you sit at a desk using a computer (or put a laptop on your lap for that matter!) with a wireless connection, you expose your chest to wireless radiation throughout the day. A safer alternative is to connect to the Internet via a wired cable to reduce wireless radiation exposure to your chest. If you exercise this option, make sure Wi-Fi is turned off on your computer. The same principal applies if you use an e-reader, tablet or any other wireless devise at a table. You also don't want these devices on your lap for the same reason.

Around the home, other contributors of electromagnetic frequencies are batteries, plugs and chargers. You can use a battery operated alarm clock to keep frequencies away from your head at night. You can unplug corded chargers for toothbrushes, razors, and phones while you are home and plug them in while you are away.

If you live near power lines, transmitters or towers, you may have higher electromagnetic frequencies in your home. Old power lines can cause some frequencies to travel through land, so being near a pond, river or pool can increase frequencies around the home. Plug in style filters can be used on the outlets in your home to decrease EMF, but can be expensive to install. To find out if EMFs are an issue in your home's outlets, you can buy a test meter at www.stetzerelectric.com for about $125.

Our goal here is to keep radiation exposure at a minimum as much as possible. The breast cancer danger comes from the total cumulative dose of radiation on your body, especially the chest area over time.

Conclusion

We can see that there are re-occurring methods for reducing these seven categories of external proestros. It may not be too difficult, after all, to eradicate the high risk proestros out of our life by following these tips:

1) Filter house water
2) Check labels on personal care products and foods
3) Use homemade cleaners and natural pesticide products
4) Use glass or ceramic cookware, food and water storage
5) Rinse fruit and vegetables
6) Buy wax paper wrapped cheese products
7) Wash hands after using electrical equipment and keep equipment a safe distance from the body

How to Eradicate Water Contaminants

Since your home's water supply is what gives your body the water of life and filtering your water keeps these proestros down, I researched water filtration in order to help you make this very important decision. Your body is made up of 99% water (or at least hydrogen and oxygen), so you can see why water is really important! There are so many different contaminants that can be in water. Summarizing what we have reviewed thus far, contaminants are classified as halides (chlorine and fluoride), microbiological (cysts, bacteria, parasites), radiological contaminants (arsenic, lead, copper, aluminum, mercury, radon and asbestos) and lastly, Volatile Organic Compounds (VOCs), which include chemicals, pesticides, herbicides, insecticides, hormones, PCBs, trihalomethanes (THMs) all of which are by-products of chlorination.

If you are on a public water system, you may need to filter out chlorine, fluoride and THMs. They are not good to put on your body, your skin or to drink. On the periodic table of elements, chlorine and fluoride are in the same class as iodine and may take up receptor sites for iodine in your breast, thyroid and ovaries.

Whether you are on well or public water, it is a good idea to make sure you are filtering out endocrine disrupters such as pesticides and herbicides. Here is what Linda S. Birnbaum, Ph.D., DABT, ATS, Director, National Institute of Environmental Health Sciences said about endocrine disrupting chemicals in water in 2010:

"Over the past fifty years, researchers observed increases in endocrine-sensitive health outcomes. Breast and prostatic cancer incidence increased between 1969 and 1986; there was a four-fold increase in ectopic pregnancies (development of the fertilized egg outside of the uterus) in the U.S. between 1970 and 1987; the incidence of cryptorchidism (undescended testicles) doubled in the U.K. between 1960 and the mid-1980s; and there was an approximately 42% decrease in sperm count worldwide between 1940 and 1990."
These chemicals are known to affect animals when they enter the water supply as well." [375]

Make no mistake; these substances are contributing to unhealthy bodies, but you don't have to buy an expensive whole house filter. You can get separate filters for your sink faucet, shower and/or refrigerator if you want to keep costs down. Here are options for filters:

Bottled water

Bottled water has started falling out of popularity lately for several reasons. Chemicals such as BPAs from plastic bottles can leech into the

---

[375] Linda S. Birnbaum, Ph.D., DABT, ATS Director National Institute of Environmental Health Sciences, National Institutes of Health, Director, National Toxicology Program February 25, 2010 *Endocrine Disrupting Chemicals in Drinking Water: Risks to Human Health and the Environment.*

water, on top of the fact that bottled water costs more and is a major source of waste. In most cases, the water itself is no different than tap water. Filtering your house water is the least expensive option. For these reasons, it is not a good idea to buy bottled water if you can help it. Nestle's® bottled water was rated the highest by Dr. Joseph Mercola's website for purity and due to the fact that Nestle discloses its sources of water and additives. It is the only one I buy if I am traveling where I'll need bottled water. As another alternative, I save glass milk bottles and reuse them for water to take on trips.

Pitcher and faucet water filters

Pitcher water filters like Brita and Clear2O use charcoal granules to remove contaminants. They are less expensive than other filter options upfront, but require frequent filling and cartridge replacement (making them more expensive in the long run). Faucet mount filters also use charcoal to remove contaminants. Faucet mount filters cannot be used with hand held or pull out style faucets, which limits their use since many new faucets are this style.

Charcoal filters claim to reduce chlorine, lead, copper, toluene, mercury, cadmium, zinc and some organics but are not effective at removing all VOCs, pesticides, herbicides or fluoride. Even though claims are made about reducing lead, Consumer Reports reported in February 2012 that Brita does a poor job at it. This is the reason they didn't even compare Brita in their evaluation that year.

Overall, pitcher and faucet mount filters improve water taste, are better than no filter at all, but not the best option for the task of reducing all proestros.

Refrigerator filters

Newer refrigerator filters are actually pretty good. Whirlpool makes a two-stage filter (also for Kenmore, Kitchen Aid, Maytag, Amana and Jenn-Air side by side refrigerators) that claims to remove particulates,

VOCs, parasites, pesticides and herbicides, asbestos, chemicals, lead, mercury and chlorine. One stage encompasses the carbon filter and the other stage includes ionization. The only substance not filtered is fluoride. If you are on well-water, fluoride will most likely not be in your water. The filters sold under the Whirlpool name seem to be less expensive, so those would be the better option if you decide to go with a refrigerator filter.

Reverse osmosis (RO) filter

Reverse osmosis filtration utilizes a membrane that removes many contaminants from water. It is usually paired with a granule charcoal filter to remove chlorine. It is typically installed at your main water line for the entire house and has to be installed by a plumber, which adds to the up-front cost. It can also be mounted under the kitchen sink for filtration of this fixture only.

The semi-permeable membrane separates many contaminants (which usually have a larger particle size than water) and rejects a large amount of water in the process. Because of this, it may reduce water pressure while in use. It takes up to an hour to filter one gallon of water. Reverse osmosis wastes several gallons of water for every gallon filtered and many naturally occurring minerals (including calcium and magnesium) are also removed from the water.

Reverse osmosis does reduce arsenic, fluoride, asbestos, and heavy metals. It does not filter VOCs or some proestros like pesticides and herbicides. Filters need to be replaced regularly and they are costly. RO does remove a large amount of contaminant but since we are specifically looking to get rid of VOCs, pesticides and endocrine disrupters, along with chlorine, they may not be worth the inconvenience of low water pressure and upfront and ongoing cost.

Distilled water

The distillation process uses heat to turn water into steam. The steam rises and moves to a cooling chamber where it turns back into liquid, leaving behind many contaminants. This process reduces large particles like minerals and heavy metals, arsenic, asbestos and fluoride but does not remove pesticides or herbicides or VOCs. It does effectively kill bacteria. Long term use can cause mineral deficiencies.

Home distillation systems do exist, but they are large and expensive and cannot be used during a power outage. Although this process removes many contaminants, it is costly and still doesn't remove everything we need it to, especially pesticides and VOCs!

Solid block carbon filters

Solid block carbon filters are recognized by the EPA as the best option for removing chemicals like herbicides, pesticides and VOCs. They are typically installed on the counter top or below the sink. Quality carbon block filters will also remove chemicals, bacteria, fluoride, heavy metals, nitrate, nitrites and parasites. Most solid block filters are gravity based and, amazingly, can safely transform any type of water into safe drinking water including rain water and pond water. Since these filter VOCs, heavy metals, chlorine, fluoride, nitrates/ites, bacteria, parasites, herbicides, pesticides, chemicals and VOCs, it is the best performing option for breast cancer prevention. The filter only needs to be changed approximately every six months. It also doesn't require electricity or water pressure to work, so is operational during a power outage. There are two subclasses of solid block carbon filters. One type is a lower cost and last three years and the other lasts up to ten years.

One brand of carbon block filter I found online is the Aquasana, two or three stage filters. Aquasana's products use multiple processes to filter water. One cartridge uses a filter media which filters out the larger sediment. The other uses a carbon block to filter out more difficult contaminants. Aquasana makes shower head filters, counter top and under counter versions. The over counter unit price is a little lower priced at $86. It attaches to your sink faucet and requires pressure in order to operate. The under counter version was $171 at the time of this writing and also requires pressure to operate.

Consumer Reports rated Shaklee's *BestWater MTS 20000* countertop brand as its "Best Buy" in Feb 2012. It is priced around $260, even though it lacks a filter life indicator and has a slower flow rate than other counter top models.

Another option I've heard a lot about is the Berkey system. Berkey has a travel filter and several countertop sizes. They range from 1.7 to 4 gallons. The upfront cost is higher ($205 to $339) but there are so many advantages, it seems worth it if you can afford it. This system does not require attachment to your faucet or water pressure, so in the unlikely event of power or water disruption, it will still operate.

There are a couple of downsides to this type of filter. One is that you have to fill the tank by hand regularly. I have not evaluated the flow rate on these, but have read that most carbon block filters will have a slower flow rate, which is another down side. The other issue is that it takes up a significant amount of counter space. I have the Berkey sport bottle/portable option that I use while traveling. It uses pressure from your hand, so there is no problem with flow rate. It costs $18 at www.amazon.com or www.infowars.com.

Solid block carbon filters don't remove naturally occurring minerals from the water, making it the best tasting filtered water option. Whether you are on a well or public water, the solid block carbon filter will work great. Since I am on a well and do not need to worry about chlorine and fluoride, I chose to just use the refrigerator filter on my fridge and the travel Berkey while I am traveling.

As an aside, you may have heard about hormones in the water supply due to birth control pills making their way back in to the environment. Synthetic hormones come from various sources including ingesting "the pill" or from cattle. However, there is no scientific evidence to support the fact that "the pill" is working its way back into surface water or city drinking water. It is either non-existent or negligible.[376]

---

[376] Aug 2011 Association of Reproductive Health Professionals, Contraception

There has been some evidence of hormones making their way back into ground water via septic systems and then into well-water. A study in 2006 showed a 6 to 30-fold increase of organic wastewater contaminants in ground water to include steroid hormones 17beta-estradiol (E2) and estrone (E1), along with their glucuronide and sulfate conjugates in Cape Cod Maine. Septic tanks and underground water was tested and compared.[377] Since 25% of people in the US have a septic system, it would be a good idea to use a solid block carbon filter on your water system if you also have a well. The septic can contaminate your well-water without you realizing it.

There are a lot more compounds in water that cause endocrine disruption than any amounts found from "the pill". Your kidneys and liver are your natural filters for hormones and patentable hormones. Decreasing as many proestros contributors as possible will ease the burden for your body.

Editorial
[377] Swartz CH et al. Aug 15 2006 *Environ Sci Technol* "Steroid estrogens, nonylphenol ethoxylate metabolites, and other wastewater contaminants in groundwater affected by a residential septic system on Cape Cod, MA".

Chapter 16

P is for PROGESTERONE SUPPLEMENTATION

Like most men say, women are complicated! Well, it's true. We have so many hormones it's almost impossible to count them all. But we do need to understand some of them, if we want to understand why we need to use progesterone cream as part of being proactive against breast cancer. Progesterone, estrogen, estriol, and 2-hydroxyestrone are among the vital sex hormones to understand and will be discussed here.

By now, you will have seen how many breast cancer risk factors you have by using the table and if you may have symptoms of estrogen dominance by reviewing the lists. If so, you may be low in progesterone. You can either test your hormones before you get started taking progesterone cream, or you can test later to determine if you are on the right dose. Using progesterone cream only takes a few seconds per day, as it is applied just like lotion.

Progesterone was a miracle for me. It made everything better: PMS symptoms stopped, acne disappeared, and sex drive returned. Remember, natural progesterone activates the p53 cancer protective gene too! Eventually, I had to stop using progesterone cream, but it was the miracle that got my body back on track.

Hormone Reality Check: A HOST of DEFINITIONS

I found it interesting that terminology has gotten blurred when describing hormones. Some words are used interchangeably where they should not. This is why it is important to understand the difference between hormone-like molecules and actual hormones. Understanding this difference will help you identify what you are actually taking, ingesting and applying. There are the three different kinds of hormones in existence today.

Natural hormones are the hormones that exist naturally in human bodies, animals or plants. They exist in nature. There are no changes to them at the molecular level. A hormone is naturally produced in our body by an organ (i.e. ovaries or thyroid) and each hormone has a regulatory job within the activity of certain organs.

One classification of hormones is the *sex steroids*. In our bodies, hormones *produce* or turn into other hormones. For instance, sex hormones can turn into other non-sex steroids, like glucocorticoids. These are the main natural human sex hormones:

Estrone
Estriol
Estradiol
2-hydroxyestrone
16-hydroxyestrone
2-methoxyestrone
2-hydroxyestradiol
16-hydroxyestradiol
2-methoxyestradiol
FSH
DHEA
Testosterone
Dihydrotestosterone
Progesterone
Pregnenolone

An example of a natural animal hormone is a type of estrogen present in horses called equilin. This natural hormone is what is used in the prescription drug *Premarin*. For humans, this is a proestro for the uterus, where it promotes estrogens.

Natural hormones in plants are called phytoestrogens. Generally, plant hormones act weaker in the human body than horse hormones. They are 500 to 1000 times less active and, in general, are not considered proestros.

Bioidentical hormones are molecules that are the exact same structure as the natural hormones they are trying to imitate. It is impossible to tell them apart physically, they behave the same, and the body processes them the same as natural molecules. Bioidentical hormones are typically derived from a vegetable source such as Mexican yam. They are man-made or synthesized to have the same structure as the hormone they are trying to replicate, so they are considered synthetic. Synthetic hormones are man-made. Bioidentical synthetic hormones are *not* proestros.

Patentable hormones are not found in nature. They are really not hormones at all. Here, natural molecules are chemically tweaked so that the molecular structure differs from those found in nature so that the new structure can be patented. These are also generally referred to as *synthetic hormones* or *synthetic patentable hormones*. Most, if not all patentable hormones, have been proven at some level to act as proestros somewhere in the body.

Knowing the differences in how hormones are defined, we can now begin to understand how patentable, natural and bioidentical progesterones and estrogens function in terms of breast cancer prevention.

OUR NATURAL HORMONES

Progesterone and Estrogen

Natural estrogen and progesterone oppose each other for a balanced hormone system. Progesterone is a steroid hormone that regulates nearly every bodily function. Among its many roles, it supports gestation in pregnancy and creation of the embryo. What this translates to is that progesterone plays an important role in egg making and supporting the environment for the egg.

While John R. Lee, M.D. acknowledged the functions progesterone plays in supporting gestation and the menstrual cycle, his research revealed that this hormone plays a far greater number of roles than most doctors realize. One of those roles is controlling the proliferation of cells throughout the body, including the reproductive system and the breasts. For instance, one of progesterone's roles is to stop the growth of cells that line the uterine walls prior to menstruation. This means that progesterone plays an important role in opposing estrogen, preventing, and stopping breast cancer from spreading. Dr. Lee described estrogen and progesterone's role in regards to cell growth in his book, *What Your Doctor May Not Tell You About Breast Cancer*:

"In breast tissue, estrogen stimulates breast duct cells to proliferate, whereas progesterone inhibits this proliferation and causes maturation and differentiation of the cells, making them more resistant to cancerous changes. Breast duct cell proliferation is considered to be an early sign of the changes that lead to breast cancer."

When the body is out of balance with estrogen or progesterone, there are many physiological effects that can take place. Following, is a list of those effects as presented by Dr. John R. Lee, MD.

Table Index

* Indicates that those effects are caused by estrogen dominance, or an imbalance of estrogen caused by too little progesterone.
** Indicates that these effects are caused by an excess of progesterone.
*** Indicates that these effects are caused by a deficiency of estrogen.

Reprinted by permission of The Official Website of John R. Lee, M.D.

PHYSIOLOGICAL EFFECTS OF ESTROGEN AND PROGESTERONE

Estrogen Effects

Progesterone Effects

Estrogen Effects	Progesterone Effects
Creates proliferative endometrium	Maintains secretory endometrium
Breast cell stimulation (fibrocystic breasts *)	Protects against breast fibro cysts
Increased body fat and weight gain*	Helps use fat for energy
Salt and fluid retention	Natural diuretic
Depression, anxiety, and headaches*	Natural anti-depressant and calms anxiety
Cyclical migraines	Promotes normal sleep patterns
Poor sleep patterns	Facilitates thyroid hormone function
Interferes with thyroid function*	Helps normalize blood sugar levels
Impairs blood sugar control*	Normalizes blood clotting
Increased risk of blood clots*	Helps restore normal libido
Little or no libido effect*	Normalizes zinc and copper levels
Loss of zinc and retention of copper*	Restores proper cell oxygen levels
Reduced oxygen level in all cells*	Prevents endometrial cancer
Causes endometrial cancer*	Helps prevent breast cancer1
Increased risk of breast cancer*	Decreased risk of prostate cancer
Increased risk of prostate cancer*	Stimulates new bone formation
Restrains bone loss	Improves vascular tone
Reduces vascular tone (dilates blood vessels)	Prevents autoimmune diseases
Triggers autoimmune diseases*	Increases sensitivity of estrogen receptors
Creates progesterone receptors	Necessary for survival of embryo
Relieves hot flashes***	Precursor of corticosteroid biosynthesis
Prevents vaginal dryness and mucosal atrophy***	Prevents coronary artery spasm and atherosclerotic plaque
Increases risk of gall bladder disease*	
Improves memory***	
Improves sleep disorders***	Sleepiness and depression**
Improves health of urinary tract***	Digestive problems*
Relieves night sweats***	

Estriol and 2-Hydroxyestrone are Not Proestros

Progesterone is not the only hormone that can keep cell proliferating estrogens in check. It turns out the estrogen called estriol, can also do it. Many women having menopausal symptoms can take estriol as a cream and manage symptoms without increasing the risk of breast cancer.

Estrogens like estriol and 2-hydroxyestrone are not cell promoters. Science has found that a large percentage of women diagnosed with estrogen related cancer (i.e. breast and ovary) are low in 2-hydroxyestrone and high in 16-hydroxyestrone.[378] 16-hydroxyestrone is a cell promoter. Increasing 2-hydroxyestrone and decreasing 16-hydroxyestrone lowers breast cancer risk

It is important to know the difference between the two estrogens, estriol and estradiol. Australian researchers in 1996 studied the visual effect on women's skin using estriol and estradiol. Both hormones caused improvement in firmness, elasticity, moisture content, increase in new blood vessels and a decrease in wrinkle depth and pore size by 61% to 100%. Both estrogens were equally effective, but estradiol caused more side effects.[379]

Natural Anti-Estrogen 2-Methoxyestradiol

Scientists have found ways to offset proestros by increasing anti-estrogens. One hormone in particular is showing tons of great evidence as an anti-estrogen. It inhibits cell propagating estrogens. It also inhibits the metastasis of cancer. It is 2-methoxyestradiol (2ME2). The Mayo Clinic is performing clinical trials on a pill form. Even though this is a natural hormone, the press release on this study called it an estrogen derived drug, even though it already exists naturally in our bodies.

---

[378] Annie Im et al. Sep 2009 *Carcinogenesis* "Urinary estrogen metabolites in women at high risk for breast cancer".
[379] Schmidt JB et al. Sep 1996 *Int J Dermatol* "Treatment of skin aging with topical estrogens".

Scientists made some progress with 2ME2 in the Mayo Clinic study because instead of delivering the hormone orally, which is not good for the liver or as effective, they started using injections, which were more effective. What a surprise! No adverse effects from doses of 200, 400, 600 or 800 mg were found. Unfortunately, there is no 2ME2 available in the market at this time, so we have to try to increase this hormone naturally. There are ways to do this, believe it or not. Supplements such as SAMe, MSM, THF and TMG (in this book's supplement section) all raise 2ME2 levels.

BIOIDENTICAL PROGESTERONE

Progesterone has been detected in at least one plant, *juglans regia*. In addition, progesterone-like substances are found in *Dioscorea* species of plants.[380] Russell Marker, a chemist from Penn State University, discovered an easy and inexpensive way to make large quantities of bioidentical human progesterone from the Mexican yam, *Dioscorea composita*. These plants contain a progesterone-like substance called diosgenin that can be taken and converted into progesterone that matches human progesterone. This is called a *bioidentical hormone*. His method of extraction, called the *Marker degradation*, was able to turn out other forms of hormones, including estrogen.

In 1944 Russell Marker started manufacturing bioidentical progesterone using his Marker degradation method. Due to his discovery of this method, other companies, such as pharmaceutical companies, starting using his Marker degradation method to manufacture patentable hormones from the same plant Marker was utilizing.

Bioidentical hormones can also be made into a pill or capsule to be put under the tongue and absorbed in the mouth. Much higher doses are

---

[380] Pauli GF et al. Mar 2010 *J Nat Prod* "Occurrence of progesterone and related animal steroids in two higher plants."

needed for oral progesterone and it works best if it is crushed into small particles or *micronized*. This process makes the progesterone particles really small so that they can bypass the stomach and liver. The only side effect known is sleepiness. Pills are not the method integrative doctors typically recommend because the body processes hormones differently through the stomach, which can end up causing digestive stress.

The proven science behind using progesterone supplementation is found in several studies. One study in 1995, called the PEPI study (Post-menopausal Estrogen-Progestin Intervention), showed there were no adverse effects associated with its use. It was the only NIH sponsored trial that tested bioidentical progesterone (in micronized pill form). This study also found that after 36 months, *Premarin*, including bioidentical progesterone, helped prevent bone loss.[381]

A more recent breakthrough study in 2015 showed that progesterone could slow or decrease breast cancer tumor cells and then the actual tumors in mice.[382] These studies confirm the conclusions made by John R. Lee, M.D. and David Zava, Ph.D. about progesterone over a decade ago. The most interesting part of what this latest study shows is that progesterone causes progesterone receptors to attach themselves to estrogen receptors and once they do that, estrogen receptors stop turning on genes that promote cancer cell growth! Not only did they turn off estrogen receptors, they also turned on genes that promote the death of cancer cells and growth of normal cells. These studies were performed first in cells and then on mice for only 25 days with treatment of both progesterone and estrogen. The tumors in mice *decreased* in size after only 25 days! Imagine if they'd *only* given them progesterone!

---

[381] The Writing Group for the PEPI trial 1995 *JAMA* "Effects of estrogen/progestin regimens on heart disease risk factors in post-menopausal women" The Post-Menopausal Estrogen/Progestin Interventions (PEPI) Trial.
[382] Perks Bea July 2015 *Pharmaceutical Journal* "Progesterone receptor could slow breast cancer growth".

Cellular and animal studies have not been the only way to prove bioidentical human hormones work. Doctors putting thousands of women on bioidentical hormones since the 1980s, is also proof. No problems have ever been reported for hundreds of thousands of women who have used bioidentical progesterone cream, including myself. In addition, the risks of proper use of bioidentical hormones has never been documented by the pharmaceutical industry or anyone for that matter. Well, the reality is that genuine bioidentical hormones are the same as human hormones and those have been present in our bodies since our existence!

A Patentable Hormone: PROGESTIN

Progestin was first developed in the 1950s and marketed in the US by Parke-Davis in 1957 as *Norlutin*. It was used in some of the first oral contraceptives in the early 1960s. Some examples of progestins that have been used in hormonal contraceptives since then are norethynodrel (Enovid), norethindrone, norgestimate, norgestrel, levonorgestrel, medroxyprogesterone, desogestrel, etonogestrel, ethinyl estradiol and drospirenone. I think I was on some of those drugs! These products may act like the natural hormone for the purpose they are serving, but they may also function like other hormones as a negative side effect.

In order to encapsulate the progesterone-like version of these drugs, a name was created for these patentable hormones. They called them *progestins* or *progestogens*. They are not actual hormones that exist on this planet. Birth control pills and IUDs contain progestins or a combination of natural estrogen and progestin. Since patented birth control methods have some component that is not part of our normal body, over time they contribute to the build-up of estrogen in our body, specifically in our fat cells. This is perhaps a reason why, even after menopause when natural estrogen levels decrease, women's risk of breast cancer rises. These molecules remain in the breast's fat cells.

There has been misuse between the terms progestin and progesterone by the media, pharmaceutical and medical industry. In addition, the term *hormone* has been used interchangeably for patentable hormones, including progestins. It has come to be accepted that if a molecule acts like a hormone somewhere in the body, it is a hormone. However, this is not true, they are actually molecules acting in disguise of hormones and behind the scenes they are doing damage.

For every natural human hormone, there is a corresponding enzyme or chemical that will break it down without producing toxic by-products. The human body lacks the ability to metabolize alien and non-human patentable hormones in the same way. Science has shown us that progestins may oppose patentable estrogens, but science does not tell us that the body excretes progestins naturally.

In a review in 2006, Yager and Davidson state that *"progestins tend to increase cell proliferation"*, which is a known mechanism for carcinogenesis.[383] Progestins are transformed into testosterone, which in turn, transforms into estrogen. Progestins increase cell division where natural progesterone does not. Watson Laboratories, Inc., a manufacturer of a pill form of natural progesterone, stated in 2013 that there is no increased risk of breast cancer with progesterone supplementation.

If you look on the labels of your prescription hormone drugs, you may even see the prescriptions being called progesterone or estrogen. You may also see it in studies. The fact is, they are not progesterone or estrogen. These are patentable hormones and are proestros. They generally increase estrogen somewhere in our bodies! Understanding the difference between real-natural, bio-identical and synthetic patentable hormones, will enable you to make logical choices when it comes to patentable hormones and breast cancer prevention.

---

[383] Yager JD and Davidson NE Jan 2006 *N Engl J Med* "Estrogen Carcinogenesis in Breast Cancer".

HISTORY OF SYNTHETIC PATENTABLE HORMONES

When we start to go into menopause, which can be anywhere from late 30s to mid-40s, progesterone and/or estrogen production decreases. Many women get menopausal symptoms such as hot flashes, memory loss and night sweats. Because of these symptoms, in the 1920s, a couple of American and German scientists actually developed pills that used human hormones to resolve menopausal symptoms. The problem arose when they had to collect urine from pregnant women for this pill. The pills still had a urine odor and taste, so it was not very marketable. Due to this unfortunate experience, pharmaceutical companies strayed away from using human urine to relieve symptoms, even though this would have been a safer alternative to the drugs we use today.

In the 1970s pharmaceutical companies developed an estrogen product made from horse urine because it was easier to collect. Horse hormones are nothing like human hormones, they are not molecularly the same and they act differently in the human body. Since the human body does not have all the enzymes needed to break down horse hormones, residues of this type of hormone can build up in the liver over time.

One of these estrogen products goes by the name of *Premarin,* which stands for pregnant mare's urine. Isn't it nice to know we are ingesting horse urine? The companies that put this pill together realized quickly that supplementing with unopposed natural horse estrogen caused uterine and endometrial cancer, so they decided to create *Provera,* a synthetic, patentable version of progesterone. *Provera* has turned out to be extremely carcinogenic, but is still FDA approved. *Provera* was used to oppose horse estrogen to prevent endometrial cancer, which was successful. But, as you read before, using this combination caused a significant increase in breast cancer. So even though *Provera* stopped uterine cancer, it promoted breast cancer. Usually, if a substance is known to have deadly side effects, it is taken off the market. However, in this case, the manufacturer for *Provera* lowered the dose hoping that the side effects would not be as bad. This new FDA approved pill is called *Prempro*. It was evidently approved without further studies on its link to breast cancer.

Having realized that horse urine is not well received or tolerated, many companies developed a third type of drug. A natural/synthetic combination called *Prefest* or *ClimaraPro*. Knowing that progesterone opposes estrogen, they used natural human estrogen and combined it with synthetic progestin. Since there was at least one patentable hormone in the mix, they could still patent the pill. Still, the problem here is that progestins don't expel out of the body properly and actually do not have the same opposing effect on all or some estrogens.

In addition, since most progestins are in pill form and ingested, they get bogged up in the liver. Taking any hormones by mouth distorts their natural metabolism. First, they have to make it through our stomach acid and digestive enzymes. Any that survive this, are absorbed in the small intestine and go directly to the liver. Pharmaceutical companies make progestins with high levels of hormone so they stay biologically active in the stomach and can circulate through the body. Since natural human hormones do not stay active in the stomach, a bioidentical human hormone pill cannot be used for oral contraception.

The liver acts as a screening service. It passes some onward, modifies others and rejects a few. The liver is very efficient at metabolizing and neutralizing human steroid hormones. Very little of the actual original hormone dose makes it into the bloodstream intact.

However, when alien molecules such as those made in a lab are ingested, the liver lacks enzymes to break them down efficiently. This sometimes leads to the formation of toxic metabolites that are eight times more potent than the original synthetic hormone. Your liver can be pushed to its limit with overuse of patentable hormones.

An interesting fact that I pointed out in Part I, was that from the 1940s to 1970s breast cancer incidences have climbed slowly and steadily. In the late 70s to early 80s the cancer rate among women age 45 and up went up by 300% until about 1999 when the rate leveled off. In 2003 after women stopped using horse hormones for menopause, a drop happened. Interestingly enough, the steady increase over the years in breast cancer coincides with increased use of hormonal birth control, pesticide exposure and menopausal medication, as shown in charts in Part I of this book.

Since many women started using more natural alternatives after the WHI study in 2002, pharmaceutical company manufacturers have started a battle against bioidentical hormones being produced. Pharmaceutical companies cite that if their hormones aren't safe, then the bioidentical ones are not safe either. All the case studies albeit small, in virtually every case, show that bioidentical human estrogens and progesterones are safer than *Premarin* and *Provera*. However, even natural estrogens should not be given if a person has been exposed to proestros because even too many natural estrogens can increase cell proliferation.

HOW TO USE PROGESTERONE CREAM

Now that you've read about a few of our key hormones, you can see why we are here at battle Step P, adding progesterone to our routine. Progesterone keeps all the excess estrogen stored in your body from causing cells to replicate. By this point, you will have done a saliva or urine hormone test as discussed in Part II. You will now know if you have an estrogen issue and perhaps other hormone issues that need balancing.

Hopefully, you have found a doctor that can tailor specific doses or timing to your schedule. If you have gone this far, you are likely going to be adding progesterone cream or an estriol/progesterone combination cream to your daily regimen based on your test results and age.

It is important to get a quality bioidentical hormone product. Although over the counter forms are readily available, ordering from a compounding pharmacist would ensure more accurate dosing and quality. Most women use gels or creams to apply bioidentical hormones to their skin. Through applying it this way, the hormones diffuse through the skin and go directly into the bloodstream. The hormones are then delivered directly to the heart which in turn sends them to cells all over the body.

The type of progesterone that I used is the natural, bioidentical progesterone derived from diosgenin, a saponin of the yam. It can come in a pump, squeeze tube or a container. The pumps deliver a specified dose. Squeeze tubes or pumps help to isolate the cream from contamination by the fingers. If you want to alter your dose, squeeze tubes or jars will give you that flexibility. The pumps appear to be more expensive than the jars. I started out using progesterone cream in the jar bought from this website: www.helenpensanti.com.

There are a couple of natural progesterone products that have patents due to their delivery method. *Prometrium* by Solvay Pharmaceuticals is a micronized form of progesterone derived from a plant and can be used as a suppository for women with low progesterone levels. Some women who have trouble conceiving will use this product. *Crinone* by Columbia Labs is a gel that is inserted into the vagina and is available with two different doses. This product was also made for women who are having trouble conceiving or women who do not have a period. These two products may be good alternatives to using a cream, but they are available by prescription only.

Application to the skin is one of the best ways to get hormones into your body without side effects. You can gently massage the progesterone cream into areas of thinner skin where you blush such as the neck, face, chest, inner arms or thighs, palms of the hands, or soles of the feet (unless your hands or feet are heavily callused). The optimal approach is to apply a larger dose at bedtime and a smaller dose in the morning, or as directed by your healthcare provider. If this does not work well for you, just pick one time of the day when it's most convenient to use it and apply the whole dose. Rotate areas daily to avoid saturation.

According to Doctors Wright and Lenard, the best way to apply topical creams or gels is directly to your vaginal membranes or the inner surfaces of the labia. This is most like the way our bodies deliver hormones. Natural hormones are secreted by the ovaries and are directed to the zones that would normally be receiving them. In this way, progesterone cream is acting more like our natural body. The rate of absorption is higher here and this method minimizes drowsiness, the primary side effect of excessive doses of oral progesterone.

I did not know about this method when I was using progesterone, so I never tried it. I am not sure how easy this method would be, but, don't make the mistake I did and apply it to your breasts every day. Even though it would be good to apply to the breast to help get the excess estrogen from this area, you should alternate locations. Your significant other may like the swollen side effects; however, the aching is not worth it.

Pre-menopausal women on a regular cycle or wanting to achieve a 28-day cycle will want to apply the progesterone cream 14 days prior to menses and stop two days prior to menses. Typically, this would mean you would start using the cream on day 12 of your cycle and stop on day 26 of your cycle. The cream can be started on days 10 to 15 depending on your personal cycle. Post-menopausal women can do a simulated cycle or apply it daily with a few days break at the end of 26 days.

The typical dose is 15 to 24 mgs per day. This dose can be divided up into two applications or just applied once per day. If you test really low in progesterone, you may need a higher dose. I started with 20 mg per day in two doses and went down to 15mg per day in two doses, and then 8mg once per day. I completed using it on my skin after many years. I recently tested my progesterone levels, as you saw in the urine test and my levels are fine. You can have too high progesterone after using creams for a long time, so you do want to be careful to monitor symptoms and test regularly!

Dr. Bruce Rind suggests that you can also use the cream in smaller doses starting the day after your period through day 12 and then days 24 to the start of your period based on symptoms. Again, it is best to make alterations in dosages under the consultation of a doctor. I actually applied some to my temples when I had a headache and it improved the headache within seconds!
There can be times where you may need to increase your dose if you are still having PMS or estrogen dominance symptoms. There have also been documented cases where women's symptoms do not respond to bioidentical hormone treatment. Dr. Jonathan Wright found that some women over metabolize hormones in their liver due to the excess hormones their liver is used to handling. The use of cobalt has been shown to be safe with calming an over active liver down. So, it is good to be aware if your symptoms do not go away with increased doses of progesterone. You may have an over active liver.

Regular saliva or urine hormone testing is recommended while using creams to monitor doses, since over time, the fat cells under the skin will store up enough progesterone for your body to use on its own. In time, the skin may begin to lose its ability to transmit the hormones into the bloodstream. Another route will need to be used if this is the case. You will notice high estrogen symptoms returning like sleepiness or acne if this happens. If you are very aware of your body, you may be able to tell by your symptoms if you are on the right dose.

OTHER HORMONAL TREATMENTS

Your hormone test may determine that you need to take other bioidentical hormones besides progesterone. In Part II, I reviewed DHEA, several estrogens and metabolites. Testing for free testosterone, not just total testosterone is imperative. If you are postmenopausal, you may need to get a progesterone and estriol combination cream, since estrogen levels may start to go down and menopausal symptoms may occur.

Estriol

Similar to progesterone, there is science to support using estriol as a supplement. There was a study in 1977 where 263 menopausal women took oral doses of bioidentical estriol vs. man made ethinyl estradiol. This study showed that any therapeutic dose of ethinyl estradiol caused uterine overgrowth. It also showed that bioidentical estriol was safe at a therapeutic dose.[384] A therapeutic dose means the dose in which menopausal symptoms, in this case vaginal dryness and thinning, are relieved. Uterine overgrowth did not occur with estriol until 300% to 500% higher dose was given than the therapeutic dose. That is a pretty large safety margin!

Another study in 2002 on pregnant women demonstrated that those who had higher concentrations of estriol during pregnancy had a lower risk of breast cancer 30 years later by as much as 20%.[385] So, not only is this type of estrogen safe, estriol can lower your risk of breast cancer if taken at normal levels!

Similar to progesterone, estriol is also known to impede the two other estrogens in your body, estrone and estradiol. If your estriol count is low, your risk of breast cancer goes up. Studies have been documented by a Dr. Henry Lemon, M.D. to support this. He also found in a small informal unpublished study that in 40% of women, who had breast cancer go into their bones, went into remission after taking high doses of estriol.[386]

---

[384] Hustin J and Van den Eynde JP Mar 1977 *Acta Cytologica* "Cytologic evaluation of the effect of various estrogens given in postmenopause".

[385] Siiteri PK et al. 2002 *Department of Defense Breast Cancer Research Meeting* "Prospective study of estrogens during pregnancy and risk of breast cancer."

[386] Follingstad A 1978 *JAMA* "Estriol, the forgotten estrogen?"

Some formulations of estrogen creams have high amounts of estriol and are safe. Dr. Jonathan Wright writes prescriptions for *Biest*, a bioidentical estriol cream for menopausal women.

If you are using the right cream at the right time in your cycle, there are many documented benefits, to using bioidentical hormone replacement. They include help with sleep issues, relieving depression, maintaining an acidic environment within the vagina which keeps good bacteria present against infections, reduction of hot flushes and acne, keeping skin elastic and younger looking, prevention of bone loss, maintaining HDL levels which is protective for the heart and a favorite... increase in libido.

DHEA

DHEA (dehydroepiandrosterone) is another hormone that declines with age. It is secreted by the adrenal glands and can act as a precursor to testosterone. It is known to help with libido problems, usually more than testosterone itself. A normal dose of DHEA is 15mg per day. This hormone is not cyclical so it can be applied daily. Over the counter versions are available.

Monitoring your hormones with DHEA is vital. Too much DHEA can be a bad thing. Your adrenals could stop producing hormones altogether, which could be disastrous. Dr. Joseph Mercola says many doctors believe you should take "holidays" with this hormone to make sure your adrenal glands keep producing their own hormones. He also recommends using this cream in the morning only, because that is when your body naturally produces it. Again, this cream is best administered through the epithelial membranes, as it can accumulate in the fat cells of the skin.

Progesterone and DHEA creams are available without a prescription. You certainly could try these for a few months to see how you feel, but it would be very important to get your urine or saliva tested after three months so you know how much more or less you need to use.

Estradiol Products

Companies have actually realized that bioidentical hormones, including estradiol, are utilized best by the body compared to patentable versions. Therefore, companies have made products with bioidentical hormones, and at the same time, have been able to patent them by way of the delivery method. These products need a prescription of course.

One product for postmenopausal women is called *FemRing*. It is a silicone ring placed inside the vagina that has bioidentical estradiol in it. *FemRing* is patented because of the delivery method of the ring. I read about some women having reactions to the ring itself or the size of it, being too small or too large. There is no anti-estrogen combined with it, so eventually it could cause overgrowth of cells, if not monitored properly. There are also skin patches, like *Estraderm* that deliver bioidentical estradiol.

Bioidentical estradiol is much more potent than estriol. Even at low doses, it is likely to cause unwanted side effects. The preferred way to utilize estradiol is to take it with other opposing hormones such as estriol or progesterone. Estriol, as described earlier, opposes the growth of cells. It's a good idea to stay clear of any bioidentical estradiol, unless it is given in combination with anti-estrogens and prescribed by a doctor.

Why would you want to supplement with some estrogen after we just got finished getting estrogen out of our body? Good question. The estrogens that have been accumulating in our bodies are estrogen metabolites or proestros which cause cell overgrowth. Many of these have increased in our bodies because of the contaminants in our environment and foods we eat. Many of us have also taken non-human horse estrogens or patentable synthetic hormones for birth control or therapy. These estrogenic products are not biologically the same as our natural estrogens. There are so many proestros and not enough anti-estrogens that we may need to put some real hormones in our body while we take out the bad. Out go the bad, in with the good, if you test low in estrogen!

Testosterone Products

Testosterone is available only with a prescription. Testosterone levels start to decline after menopause. Unfortunately for us, there is no widely accepted use of testosterone cream for women in the US. There is a patentable testosterone on the market, but here in the US it is not recommended by many doctors. It is an alien molecule that can have severe side effects.

The only other option if you are low in testosterone is to try and locate a compounding pharmacist who could formulate a cream with it in it. There are also testosterone skin patches and pellets for women that have been approved by insurance carriers in Europe. However, pellets do not copy nature with a monthly "break" in hormone exposure! Not following a normal cycle for a long period of time can lead to higher cancer risk.

Low testosterone levels can cause similar symptoms as low progesterone or estrogen, so that is another reason to get a hormone test. Women's bodies only need a tiny fraction (3 to 5%) of testosterone than what men need. A compounding pharmacist would be able to put a personalized combination cream together that raises low hormone levels. However, most integrative and medical doctors do not recommend that women take testosterone in any form.

Compounding Pharmacies

Before patent medicine, every pharmacist was a compounding pharmacist. In the 1930s and early 1940s, 60% of all prescriptions were made or compounded in the neighborhood pharmacy. Nowadays, pharmacists are mostly educated in counting pills. A compounding pharmacist can measure out appropriate doses and add them to a medium such as cream or gel. To make sure the patient uses the correct dose, they will put hormone formulations into small syringes. Hormone compounding is more complex and the equipment is costly.

Compounded creams are typically void of all dyes, flavorings, fillers and preservatives, but you don't have to worry, you won't be missing those. It is important to note that all the materials used by compounding pharmacies are subject to FDA inspection and the FDA's *Good Manufacturing Procedures* code. There is a voluntary accreditation for compounding pharmacies called *Compounding Accreditation Board*. It would be good to make sure the pharmacy that you choose has this seal. This gives the assurance that the pharmacy has met the highest quality and safety standards and that it is inspected by its state pharmacy board.

There may be a local compounding pharmacy nearby where you live. If not, they are accessible via the internet. Compounding pharmacies can also refer you to a doctor! To locate a compounding pharmacy, you can check out these agencies:

International Academy of Compounding Pharmacies (IACP) www.iacprx.org 800-927-4227

Professional Compounding Centers of America (PCCA) www.pccarx.com 800-331-2498

National community Pharmacists Association (NCPA)

American Pharmacists Association (APhA)

Here are a few online compounding pharmacies:

www.womensinternational.com

www.Koshlandpharm.com

www.meridianvalleylabs.com

My doctor recommends the following compounding pharmacies in Maryland and DC area:

Village Green Apothecary
Knowles Apothecary
Brookeville Apothecary

Chapter 17

PUTTING THE S.L.E.E.P. METHOD TO WORK

We, as a culture, have the ability to make a shift in the medical world. It is happening more and more as we watch people like Suzanne Somers promote bioidentical hormones and Food Babe fight to keep the food industry in check. Being armed with the knowledge of what causes most breast cancers, gives us hope which in turn, gives us the energy we need to take action. As we start to make changes with our bodies, money is driven into market places that work positively. Becoming active by telling people what is working for you, changes the way people think. It may not happen overnight, it may take decades, but I believe we can cause a cultural shift that can cause breast cancer rates to decrease. Together we can make a difference.

We've seen how breast cancer can be prevented and heard cases in which cancer has actually been cured without surgery. The point is, there are many drugs and supplements that may help cure or prevent future breast cancer. The medical industry and alternative health industries can work together to stop this disease. We don't have to choose sides.

We do have to realize that life may not always be as simple as taking one pill. We may actually have to take action in order to stay healthy. We may not be able to always rely on the medical industry to give us *the answer*. We can work with the knowledge that the medical industry gives us and armed with it, gain insight into prevention strategies that can actually work. Maybe someday there will be a medical cure, but for now, we can use the S.L.E.E.P. Method, and attack one of the major causes of breast cancer…. excess proestros.

It takes a lot of time and effort to be healthy these days and understandably, many people may not want to make that effort.

However, even if we cause a slight cultural shift by making thermograms and saliva or urine testing mainstream by their demand, people will begin to have new understanding while taking greater steps toward prevention.

Could the S.L.E.E.P. Method be a cure? There have been a few cases that show that this method slows or shrinks tumors, but unfortunately not enough documented cases at this point. Dr. Bruce Rind has personally seen parts of the S.L.E.E.P. Method reduce lump size in patients who have hormone related breast cancer. Unfortunately, the patients are not on the method long enough to determine if it can make the lump go away completely. They typically decide to have the lump surgically removed, rather than wait, even if it shows signs of shrinkage.

As you will see in the testimonials, there are women who have partially healed using this method and many breast cancer survivors who are already doing these steps to prevent recurrence. This method takes time, which some women may not have if they are diagnosed with aggressive breast cancer. A person may be able to achieve full estrogen detoxification within one year, but it may take up to three years.

That being said, there is no reason why most of the steps in the S.L.E.E.P. Method could not be used in tandem with today's breast cancer treatment protocols. Lifestyle changes, eradicating proestros and eating good food will most certainly not harm you! Using supplements and progesterone, however, should be approved by a doctor first.

These five steps, used together with one objective, provide a new methodology and protocol for breast cancer prevention. I was one of a few that have tried and tested it, to show it works. From research, testimonials and my personal experience, perhaps more than 75% of breast cancers are preventable if women would follow the five steps in the S.L.E.E.P. Method.

It is important to realize that the order in which the letters in the word S.L.E.E.P. is not necessarily the order to take action. Any order can be taken with this method. If you want to go step-by-step with goals and focus, you can do the challenge I have included next.

Whenever goals are set as part of a plan, they become achievable. Monitoring your achievement and seeing how you compare with others is motivating. Having a friend or an accountability partner are also ways to keep you motivated. In fact, I set up an interactive website where people can support each other's efforts. You can log in to see how others are doing at www.proestrofree.com!

THE SIX MONTH S.L.E.E.P. CHALLENGE

Step 1: 40 Day Testing, Planning and Lifestyle Challenge

- Take the written estrogen test, then order a hormone test.
- Consider options for non-hormonal birth control.
- Research doctors in your area that will support S.L.E.E.P. Methods. Make an appointment. Get Rx for Vitamin D lab work.
- Find a thermography testing location and make an appointment.
- Re-organize budget to add health expenses.
- Shop for new wireless bras.
- Practice lymphatic massage.
- Reverse set alarm no later than 9:30pm to force yourself to do a bedtime relaxation routine and go to bed early. During night time routine do ten minutes of prayer, meditation, listening to soft music or yoga.
- Write on calendar the days and times you will exercise. Set up two to three days per week. Download a short exercise routine like Phil Cambell's *Peak Fitness*, *21 Day Fix* by Beach Body or *Turbulence Training* by Craig Ballantyne.

Step 2: 30 Day Eradicate Proestros Challenge

- Throw away Teflon and coated pans.

- Buy new glass or ceramic water drinking bottles.
- Buy new shampoo, lotion, soap, body wash, deodorant, use the Environmental Working Group Website (www.ewg.org) to review products.
- Throw out proestro skin care products.
- Buy new ceramic pans at Walmart or discount section of Bed, Bath and Beyond or TJ Maxx.
- Buy new glass food storage containers at Costco, Bed, Bath and Beyond or TJ Maxx.
- Consider using an infrared sauna or some type of detox.
- Evaluate your house for environmental pollutants, and electromagnetic pollution. Reduce as needed.
- Research your water. Buy appropriate filtration.

Step 3: 30 Day Eat Right Challenge

- Make a grocery list for better healthy foods to buy. Buy organic top 12 by EWG.
- Slowly get off caffeine and sugar drinks.
- Read the labels on your current condiments. Find out what kind of fats they have, if they have soy, and how much sugar is in them.
- Switch to olive oil, coconut and healthier mayonnaise.
- Figure out where and what kind of bread you will buy or consider paleo, GAPS, ketogenic or Mediterranean diet.
- Go to www.eatwild.com or www.grasslandbeef.com and buy or order grass fed beef in bulk.
- Order grass fed whey protein online.

Step 4: 30 Day Supplement Challenge

- Order Vitamin D according to blood test results.
- Order Calcium-D-Glucarate, DIM, Milk Thistle Extract, Curcumin, and TMG
- Take iodine test and order topical or spray iodine as necessary

- Add one supplement every three to four days to check for any side effects before adding the next one. Go in this order: Milk thistle, vitamin D, TMG, DIM, Calcium-D-Glucarate and Curcumin.

Step 5: 40 Day Progesterone Challenge

- Order progesterone or prescription cream based on testing.
- Start applying on day 12 of your cycle if you have a 28-day cycle.
- Stop using two or three days prior to menses
- Keep a note pad next to your bed and monitor the good side effects!

STEP 3: EAT RIGHT

Dinner

For most people, deciding what to eat for breakfast and lunch is a fairly simple: a couple eggs, a protein shake, leftovers or a salad. Dinner is the hardest part of the day. It comes quickly after arriving at home after work and it involves the most prep time than any meal. Eating by 7pm is a good idea if you want to keep your weight in check, so that makes it even more difficult.

Planning for dinner is critical to good eating. That's why I came up with this list of ideas. I can easily look at the list, and pull something out of the freezer the morning of. Having the idea is half the battle. Making it is the other half. These are all pretty simple recipes to make and can be found in various cookbooks or online. There are three ideas for each night, so you have three weeks of ideas that you can intermix. To make dinner preparation a little easier, I will pull the ingredients from the pantry in advance. Using a slow cooker all day has also been the greatest blessing for dinner preparation. It is easy to throw frozen chicken in the crock pot, along with some *Amy's* mushroom bisque soup. Here are dinner menu Ideas:

Sunday Chili or Pasta Night

White Chicken Chili
Venison or Beef Chili
Turkey Meatballs w/ GF noodles, Spaghetti sauce and green beans

Monday Chicken Night

Honey Glazed Chicken Legs or Thighs (*Internal Bliss* p. 105)
Turkey Breast w/Cauliflower Garlic Mash or Broccoli and Gravy
Chicken and Feta Sausages

Tuesday Seafood Night

Coconut Fried Fish w/quinoa and Asparagus or Squash
Grilled or Pan Seared Cilantro-Lime Shrimp over lettuce or Quinoa
Crab Cakes or Chick Pea Fritters w/Wilted Spinach or lettuce
Salmon w/Capers and Bok Choy

Wednesday Crock Pot Night

Crock Pot Ribs w/homemade BBQ Sauce and Cauliflower
Crock Pot Cumin Chicken and Broccoli (*Dr. Mercola's Total Health Program* p.164)
Chicken w/ Cabbage and Carrots (Crockpot or Baked)
Chicken w/*Amy's* mushroom bisque soup and rice

Thursday Ground Beef or Venison

Taco Salad w/ cheese, tomato, romaine, avocado and salsa
Unstuffed Bell Peppers
Venison or Beef Burgers w/Guacamole Spread and Tomato (no bun) and Sweet Potato Fries

Friday Easy Night

GAPS Hazelnut Pizza or Zucchini/Portobello Mushroom Pizza w/Spinach or Basil
Omelet w/chives and Parmesan cheese
Oven Baked Marinara Chicken w/cheese and green beans

Saturday Burger or Steak Night

Venison or Beef Steaks w/Broccoli
Beef Stroganoff w/Spaghetti Squash
Beef tips and onions cooked in a crock pot with a bottle of organic red wine

Breakfast

Whey Protein Shake with cucumber and two slices apple or ½ banana or kiwi
1 Egg French Toast
2 Eggs over easy with Sausage
2 Egg Omelet with Spinach or chives and Parmesan Cheese
Pumpkin Almond Pancakes
GF Oats or Buckwheat Cereal w/tsp honey and whey protein.
Banana Almond Bread
Soft boiled eggs with butter and Sea salt
Poached eggs over spinach and ham w/hollandaise sauce

Lunch

Romaine or baby greens salad - Add one nut, meat, egg, dried or fresh fruit, cheese and dressing (Thai cucumber/peanut, BLT salad, Strawberry Almond)
Leftovers on a salad or rolled in a salad leaf
Roll up thinly sliced meat. Stuff with brie, basil, sun dried tomato and a pretzel.
Baked chicken nuggets
Tomato Soup w/grilled cheese sandwich
Fermented sauerkraut w/chicken sausages

Cabbage or romaine wraps w/cranberry and turkey meatballs w/hoisin sauce
Egg Salad

Snack

Celery or apple w/cream cheese or peanut/sunflower butter
Organic corn chips with guacamole or salsa and cheddar cheese
Crackers with Swiss cheese
Plain Greek yogurt with nuts or granola and Stevia or honey
Rice Cakes w/sunflower butter
Whey protein shake w/cucumber and frozen mango chunks
Veggie tray -Carrots, celery, tomato, peppers in Annie's ranch dip
Beet chips
Almond banana bread
Nut mix – GF pretzels, cashews with raisins, blueberries, or cranberries
Unsweetened apple sauce
Hardboiled egg w/ sea salt
Baked or pan fried apples w/cinnamon and walnuts
Kefir
Cucumbers in vinegar and onion
Korean dried seaweed
Organic popcorn
Artichokes in vinegar
Guacamole and non-GMO corn chips

FRIDGE AND PANTRY LIST

Here are items you can keep stocked in your fridge and pantry in preparation for the food ideas above.

Dairy
Almond, Cashew or Coconut Milk
Greek Yogurt
Organic Milk
Mozzarella and Cheddar (rBST free in wax if possible)

Swiss Cheese or Brie (in wax paper if possible)
Organic Eggs
Grass Fed Whey Protein Powder

Snacks
Beet Chips
Organic popcorn
Rice Cakes
Organic Corn chips
Guacamole
Organic Salsa
Soy free, gluten free crackers
Korean dried seaweed

Vegetables
Asparagus
Avocado
Organic Basil Plant
Beets
Bok Choy
Broccoli
Organic Carrots
Organic Celery
Frozen Cilantro Cubes
Cucumber
Garlic
Onion
Romaine Lettuce
Organic Red or Green Peppers
Organic Spinach
Organic butternut or spaghetti squash
Sweet Potatoes
Zucchini

Fruit
Organic apples

Clementines or oranges
Organic Strawberries
Cantaloupe
Bananas
Dried Cranberries, Raisins, Blueberries or Cherries
Prunes
Canned organic pumpkin
Organic Applesauce with no added sugar

Nuts
Sliced or Whole Raw Almonds
Whole Raw Brazil nuts
Whole Pecans
Cashews
Almond flour
Coconut flour
Hazelnut flour

Meats
Organic or Naturally Grown Chicken breast, legs or thighs
All natural pre-cooked chicken strips (hormone free)
Grass fed beef or venison steaks or ground meat
Wild caught Fish or shrimp
Chicken and feta sausages
GF uncured bacon
Oscar Meyer Select® GF hot dogs
All natural ground turkey or pork

Grains
GF Oats
Kind® Cereal
Sunrise® Cereal
Frootos® cereal
Buckwheat cereal
Udi's® GF Pizza Crust
Quinoa

Millet or *Udi's*® multigrain bread
Sorghum flour
Potato flour
Corn flour

Condiments/Other
Almond
Annie's® Cowgirl Ranch
Annie's® Raspberry Vinaigrette
Avocado oil
Just Mayo
Olive Oil
Coconut oil
Stevia or Dextrose
Vinegar
Organic Jelly
All natural peanut butter
Trader Joes® sunflower butter
Raw organic honey
Lime juice or fresh limes/lemons
Baking soda

Spice Cabinet – organic if possible

Basil
Ginger
Parsley
Cayenne
Chili Pepper
Cilantro
Cinnamon
Cumin
Curry
Garlic Powder
Nutmeg
Onion flakes

Oregano
Salt – pink or gray
Vanilla extract

Breast Poor

Now you may be worried about going to the poor house just to pay for your breast health. Paying for all these supplements and specialty foods can be downright expensive! Here are some tips for saving money so it can be put toward your health...only the most important thing on this earth.

-       If you are going to utilize the infrared sauna, you might as well buy one instead of paying for office visits.... that is, if you can fit it in your home. I bought a used one on Craig's List for $450. I would have spent $200 a month for office visits, so that purchase paid for itself in 2.5 months. Then, you can sell it again later when you are finished detoxifying.

-       The best deals for non-GMO organic food can be found at Wegmans, Wholefoods and Trader Joes and at your local farmer's market during the growing season. Wegmans has organic spinach for a great price and Trader Joe's dairy products and frozen meats are priced reasonably. I have tried cutting coupons, but it was not worth the time and money. Usually there are not many coupons for healthy grocery items anyway. ☹

-       Reduce, reduce, and reduce expenses! I was able to reduce my phone bill by signing up for Verizon Friends & Family and lowering my minutes. Later, I was able to switch phone companies. A *Consumer Reports* 2016 article says we should not be spending more than $50 per cell phone. I was able to lower mine to $40 per month.

-       As a business owner, I had to make some tough decisions in order to reduce expenses. I got rid of *efax*. Most people scan documents or use electronic signatures these days...fax is no longer needed. I got rid of an extra domain name I was holding onto and paying for annually, as well as monthly. I cancelled my internet for my *iPad*. I have Wi-Fi at home so I don't need the extra service. Too much internet!

-        Additional things I did were: found lower price car insurance; found a lower priced trash service; and downgraded my Comcast television service. All of these changes saved me a whopping $2640 per year or $220 per month! It is amazing how all the little things add up. Now we can afford some good food and supplements!

-        Paying for medical expenses and supplements is not the fun part of this whole experience, especially if you have to pay for them on your own. The most important way I have saved money throughout my healing process is by utilizing a high deductible Health Savings Account.

Now this may not work for you if you have to undergo major surgery...but for those own a business or who are just trying to prevent breast cancer, this is the way to go! Basically, you set up a health savings account that you put money into each month. So instead of paying the insurance company $600 to $900 per month, you are paying $600 of it to yourself. The payment to the insurance company is significantly lower than a regular plan. The deductibles can range from $2500 to $10,000. I picked the $10,000. The new federal medical plan has plans up to $6000.

All of the money put into the savings account can be written off on your taxes, whether you use it or not. Any extra money in the account collects interest. I try to keep ahead of the game and keep more money going in than out, so I can build up a nest egg in case I end up needing that $10K deductible.

If you have insurance through a company you work with, but you are going to doctors outside your regular medical plan, most likely insurance will not pay for any of it. In this case, you may be able to set up a Flexible Spending Account through your employer. This is a tax free money and can be used in much the same way as a Health Savings Account. I can't even tell you how many thousands of dollars this can save you!

- Ok, now I hope you are sitting down for this because this is the crazy part. I turned off my electric water heater to save money! I had a ten-year-old water heater and I noticed the meter turning like crazy as I was leaving the house one day. It took me turning off all the lights, and unplugging everything to figure out it was the water heater. That's when I decided to turn it off for a while.

I got my family on a similar shower schedule and decided to do dishes, laundry and showers for two days in a row. Then turn it off for two nights and one day, or something like that.

I also decided that in the winter, when the air is particularly dry, I didn't need to wash my hair every other day, but every three days. This saves electricity for blow drying my hair. My husband also doesn't shower but every three days (I know it may sound gross but he doesn't smell, believe or not!) So we put the same regimen for our child...a bath every three days in winter.

To sum it up, we use the water heater one or two days then turn it off for two nights and one day. We end up having it off about three days and five nights per week in winter. In between, we still have enough hot or warm water to wash some dishes and spruce up in the morning.

If you have a gas water heater or it is inconvenient to turn off your electric water heater, you can turn the temperature down. I also did this as ours was up too high anyway. The recommended temperature is 120 degrees. You can also get a timer if you have an electric water heater, which can turn it off at night. If you go out of town, you can turn it off, or in the case of a gas water heater, turn it to "vacation".

For the month of January, I estimated that we saved around $20 to $30. It may be difficult to figure out exactly how much you can save. One way is to look at the yellow sticker on your water heater. It will tell you the average cost per year. If you turn your water heater off half the time or 1/3 of the time, you can estimate your savings based on calculating half of the total.

Another way is to look at prior years. Last year was a warm winter and this year was cold but our total bill was only $10 more, so I know we saved some money! I just loooove finding ways to save money!

Hopefully this will spark some ideas to help you save money for your breast health. In the meantime, I will be posting products on my website, www.proestrofree.com. Hopefully, that will help!

Ending the S.L.E.E.P. Method

You may be wondering if we have to do all these steps indefinitely to prevent breast cancer. The answer is no. Once a follow up thermography shows no areas of concern and/or a hormone test shows hormonal balance, you have safely eliminated excess estrogen and chemicals out of your life! You will be able to stop the "S" and "P" parts of this method. It took me about two years.

I am sure you will be happy that you can stop ordering all those supplements. Some people will also be able to limit or completely eliminate progesterone supplementation. Hopefully, you will have noticed all the benefits of steps "L" "E", "E" and those will not be a challenge any longer. They are more permanent life changing steps.

For maintenance, you can use vitamin D, TMG, and/or utilize a multi-purpose supplement such as *XenoProtect* or *BreastDefend*. There will always be those sneaky little estrogens roaming around in some products. That's why it's good to stay on a maintenance dose or periodically take some of the supplements in the "S" section. I enjoy taking TMG and iodine because they give more energy. I naturally sweat while working out, so that is enough to excrete proestros, except in the winter when I use the infrared sauna about once a month.

TESTIMONIES

As of yet, there are not many people who I personally know who have completed the entire S.L.E.E.P. Method, but there are many people who already use many parts of it. For this reason, at this time, I am including testimonies of women who have utilized portions of the method in this book. Each heading points to the various aspects they have used for breast cancer prevention.

Good Food, Exercise and Prayer

Dr. Jill Carnahan – diagnosed age 25:
Dr. Jill was diagnosed with breast cancer stage 1 at 25 years of age. Then one year after treatment for breast cancer, she was diagnosed with Crohn's disease, which she attributes to the chemotherapy. She was able to completely heal using diet, exercise and prayer. Here is her testimony.

During my 3rd year of medical training at Loyola University in Chicago, I found an unusual lump in my left breast and with my husband's insistence; I proceeded to schedule an ultrasound and biopsy. Although I scheduled the tests, I was not the least concerned that this lump might signify something more serious. A few days later however, my worst nightmare was confirmed with a call from the surgeon. She said yes, despite all of the statistics against it at the age of twenty-five years old, I had invasive ductal carcinoma (i.e. aggressive breast cancer). I was devastated! This sudden news sent my very orderly world spinning as I began to process what the next 12 months would hold... several more surgeries, six rounds of aggressive chemotherapy followed by many weeks of radiation, Ugh! I literally went from doctor to patient overnight. The rest of that year was a blur as I took a leave of absence from medical school to complete this harsh treatment regimen. During this time, an important part of my plan for healing included nutritional supplementation, daily exercise, and prayer for healing. By the summer of 2002, I had officially "beaten" the cancer but nearly destroyed my body in the process. Completely bald, malnourished, and down to my lowest weight since fourteen years old, I was absolutely depleted but mentally still in the game.

Now over twelve years later, after relentless pursuit of personal healing I am currently in the best health of my life, completely free of breast cancer and 100% healed from Crohn's disease! I continue to eat an organic, whole food, gluten-free Paleo-style diet, exercise regularly, and practice my faith through prayer and meditation. It is evident that God healed my body expressly for the purpose of helping others and thus, I am committed to helping people find answers and live vibrantly through functional medicine. More than ever before, I believe that the human body can regain health if given the right tools... and I am living proof!

www.jillcarnahan.com

Thermography Testing, Supplements and Lymphatic Massage

This testimony can be found at www.curezone.com
White99:

Not only that, but he (Dr. Rind) suggested I have a thermogram and get my hormone levels checked and my estrogen was ridiculously high (was supported by the thermography which shows heat levels in your breasts). He gave me 2 vitamins to take and told me to do breast massages and 3 months later, my estrogen had decreased tremendously (numbers don't lie and neither does the screen that I saw with my own eyes), and continues to do so. Essentially, he prevented me from getting breast cancer.

Birth Control Pill, Exercise, Good Food

Belinda Jacobsen-Loele: diagnosed in late 40s:
I was diagnosed with invasive breast cancer five years ago and after surgery and receipt of the pathology report, the cancer was identified as a stage 1 tumor, estrogen positive. My doctor told me that a lumpectomy would not work so a mastectomy was required. I had no

history of breast cancer or lumps. Tamoxifen was used for first two years post op. Rumidex was used for the last 3 years, but this past year caused bladder and kidney issues, so it was discontinued. Note: There is a big controversy as to how long the hormonal therapy should be continued. Some doctors believe it should be ten years.

One of the things I do to avoid a recurrence of breast cancer is run (jog) and work out at the gym. The exercise gives me strength, stamina and plenty of Vitamin D. I also eat as "organic" as I can afford and buy "natural" products. I particularly work on reducing sugar intake and limiting soy (this was a big one for me being estrogen positive), GMOs, BPAs, and rBST hormones. I eat little to no processed foods and frozen dinners, or McDonald type quick food. I do not drink soda! I no longer drink milk and use unsweetened almond milk for breakfast which has more calcium and no GMOs. For the past year (year 4) I've added hemp seed hearts to my diet for added protein since I have to minimize the intake of soy and soy products which is considered plant estrogen.

I was on birth control for over 20 years but have been birth control free since June 2009. Given no family history, I believe stress and the birth control pills caused my breast cancer. There were a lot family concerns at the time I was diagnosed, but I should not have been on birth control pills for so long. I believe my GYN doctor made a mistake by extending the prescription. I also believe that my exercise program and positive attitude will continue to serve me well in years to come. ☺

Exercise, Supplements and Good Food

Patricia Reniere – diagnosed age 50:
My name is Patricia Reniere, I am 55 years old and I was diagnosed with breast cancer in September of 2010. I went in for a routine check-up and my doctor found a lump in my left breast and my pelvic exam revealed an enlarged uterus. I was sent for a mammogram and pelvic sonogram, both revealed masses. My breast mass was positive for cancer. I was diagnosed with left breast invasive mammary carcinoma

with ductal and lobular stage 11B, T2N1MO: Estrogen receptor positive Her-2-neu.

I underwent a partial mastectomy and sentinel lobe biopsy. Tumor size 2.5 cm. Nodes 1 positive. I received six rounds of chemotherapy TC averaging one treatment every six weeks. This was followed by six weeks of radiation therapy with five treatments per week. Hindsight is 20/20 as I had actually found the lump three years earlier and was sent for mammogram. I was told it was nothing to worry about. My advice to any woman is to always get a second opinion.

My type of cancer is estrogen driven. This type of cancer lives and grows with the help of estrogen. After completion of chemotherapy and radiation, it was recommended that I undergo a hysterectomy to keep the production of estrogen at bay. I began taking Femara which is a drug to help reduce the production of estrogen in the body. It was recommended that I keep taking Femara for 10 years and undergo genetic testing. I have an Ashkenazi Jewish background and the young age at which I was diagnosed put me at risk. My doctor also believed that I had the breast cancer for quite some time due to the size of the lump, my history of skin cancer and pre-cancerous colon polyp. I do have some side effects from the medicine such as intense hot flashes, bone thinning, muscular pain and stage 2 osteoporosis.

To help combat a reoccurrence I undergo routine complete blood counts, automated chemistry studies, bones scans, other testing, and personal therapies which include walking, drinking water, turmeric, a multivitamin, omega 3s, no soy, no GMOs, and I try to eat natural foods with little or no preservatives.

Supplements, Good Food, Positive Mind, Meditation, Exercise, and Breast Feeding

Lindy Liscomb - age 45 mother of three girls, Luray, VA:
I have a family history of breast cancer. I personally have been blessed with good health and have not had any issues with my breasts. I have

used birth control pills for about 15 years on and off, but not for the last 15 years.

I do not believe in self breast exams because the law of manifestation. This law says that what you look for you shall eventually find. For this reason, I also do not support any breast cancer awareness fads or organizations. I feel these increase cancer among our populations.

I believe my food is my medicine and also am aware that my thoughts, feelings and my lifestyle affect my health directly and from day to day. I am careful what I think, I do my best to follow a simple wholesome lifestyle. I do mostly walking meditations, but do sometimes sit and meditate whenever possible.

I try to eat the purest foods and supplements in a calm setting whenever possible. I rarely eat out at commercial food places as it usually is low quality and affects my health immediately. I do not consume any unnatural foods, including refined sugar, nor any fake sweeteners. I do not consume any soy or soy products with the exception of occasional consumption of fermented soy sauce.

I do my best to get as much sunlight on my body during good weather, and sometimes sunbathe during summer months; never with any sun screens! I try my best to get all the sun exposure that I can all year long.

I use coconut oil for almost all my moisture needs on my body and I only use organic products for hair/beauty products, which is very minimal.

I do not use a microwave oven, nor hair dryer.

I rarely consume any drinks or foods from plastic containers, nor do I use any Teflon or Teflon products, but only stainless steel and cast iron pans and pots.

I have done 11 liver flushes and counting, and feel this has really given me a health boost (www.curezone.com see liver flush forum).

I stopped wearing wired bras back in the 1990s and only wear camisole-type shirts under my over shirt, or no bra at all. On occasion, I will wear non-wired bras.

I also breast-fed all three of my daughters until they were past two years old. This has hopefully increased my breast health.

I live an active lifestyle where exercise is naturally incorporated in daily activities. I jump on a trampoline rebounder several times per week to increase lymph drainage, and clearing of the thoracic duct. I am very physically active.

The supplements I take currently, on top of whole unprocessed foods are:

Vitamin D from SUN and whole raw milk from my own grass-fed cow (vitamin K2 and vitamin A)
Curcumin
Iodine (30 drops per day directly on my ovaries)
Calcium (via chia seeds)
Zinc
Magnesium oil (transdermally, only)
Reishi mushroom
Shilajit
Phytoplankton

Thank you.

Bioidentical Hormones

Suzanne Somers age 60 something:
From where I sit now-calm, sane, happy, healthy, blissfully enjoying life minute by minute, enjoying the loving relationship with my husband- I am here to tell you that I found my answer with bioidentical hormones and have never looked back! Finding REAL natural bioidentical

hormones to replace my almost nonexistent ones changed the course of and quality of my life, as well as my work and life's mission. [387]

---

[387] p 140 *I'm Too Young For This*

Chapter 18

OUR FUTURE

The Future of Gene Repair

As you can see in the example of HER2 way back in Part 1, modern medicine has come up with the ability to block growth promoting proteins of genes by gene targeting. This methodology has sprouted identification of many defective cancer genes and gene targeting drugs to go along with them. Not only can drugs stop these defective genes from occurring, but scientists have found a way to actually repair broken genes. More recently, scientists have identified yet another receptor on the surface of activated T cells known as PD-1 (programmed cell-death receptor). This receptor is activated by healthy cells to make sure that the immune system doesn't harm healthy tissue. Cancer cells disguise themselves by making a lot of PD-1 to keep the immune system from attacking them.

There are new medications such as MK-3475 or *Keytruda* that specifically trigger the PD-1 to be shut down.[388] This allows the natural immune system to attack the tumor. When used in combination with other antibody drugs, clinical trials are having success rates of 85% survival with melanoma patients. Only 8% of patients experienced side effects in another study. This drug is now FDA approved for melanoma treatment and there are current clinical trials under way for 30 other types of cancers. *Keytruda* is not cancer specific because all cancers produce these antibodies.

Preliminary data for *Keytruda* with breast cancer shows that 33% of patients have shrinkage of tumors and 18.5% response rate overall for

---

[388] Estel Grace Masangkay *Clinical Leader* Dec 2014 "Merck Posts Keytruda Data in Triple Negative Breast Cancer".

triple negative breast cancer (one of the most aggressive forms of breast cancer) in patients who test positive for PD-1 proteins. Most of these patients had undergone chemotherapy which can lower immunity. I suspect better results could be obtained with patients who have fully functioning immune systems which would enable their bodies to combat the cancer. Hopefully soon, this drug will be approved for all cancers.

There is another drug targeting the same PD-1 protein called *Opdivo*. It was just FDA approved December 2014 for melanoma cancer treatment. It is a fully humanized antibody which may have better results than *Keytruda* because it is more human-like. Still both of these new drugs come with side effects.[389]

It sure would be nice to have something *now* that does not have side effects and shows a better response to cancer treatment. Well, there is a doctor located in Houston, TX who has been studying genes on another level and has had some success. Dr. Stanislaw Burzynski has found a parallel immune system in our genes (similar to the oncogenes that protect against cancer). These genes in our body protect us against cancers that float around in our body all the time (part of our immune system). As we age, or as we come into contact with various chemicals, virus and bacteria, these protective genes can be turned off by these triggers. Scientists do know what some of these triggers are. As it relates to breast cancer, scientists have discovered several genes that trigger off when a person has breast cancer. Dr. Burzynski has developed antineoplastons that work on close to one hundred genes to turn their anti-cancer effects back on.

There are over two thousand genes involved in cancer and cancer can be cured or made dormant by using just a few of them. In fact, there are twenty-four FDA approved drugs on the market that target one gene each. As you can see from modern medical studies of genes, these drugs are not always successful individually at getting rid of the cancer

---

[389] Stanberry, Porter Nov 2014 "The Next Big Step Forward for Cancer Treatment".

because only one gene is targeted, although some may reduce tumor size. However, by utilizing multiple gene targeting drugs at low doses simultaneously like Dr. Burzynski and other doctors, tumors are much more responsive.

In his practice, Dr. Stanislaw Burzynski first does testing on his patients to identify the genes that are turned off and then uses antineoplastons, along with the FDA approved gene targeted drugs and scientifically proven supplements, to turn them back on. For a patient who has defective genes that match the available drugs, over 85% have tumors that shrink or disappear completely. He typically sees a change within roughly three to four months of starting therapy.

Dr. Stanislaw Burzynski found a way to cure 58% of breast cancer patients without any side effects. He patented his treatment and years later the FDA filed thirteen copycat patents. If you have been diagnosed with breast cancer that is most likely not induced by proestros, then you might try looking into his antineoplaston therapy. In order to be part of the trials, a person must have had breast cancer and undergone chemotherapy. There are no side effects of using this drug. However, the cost will not be paid for by your insurance company.

Breast Politics

If we want to make a difference for breast cancer's future, we may need to understand breast politics. I never thought I would say those two words together, however, this day and age you turn a corner and policy is staring you in the face. Unfortunately, we may find that both natural and scientific articles can be one-sided when it comes to showing the details. Scientific articles will disclaim natural products and natural product articles will disclaim scientific research, with neither substantiating the opposing view.

Common sense tells us there are five stages with breast cancer: prevention, detection, diagnosis, treatment and cure. Research dollars are typically invested in detection, diagnosis and treatment, but not necessarily on prevention and cures. If cures became commonplace, treatment with chemotherapy drugs and radiation would not be necessary. Political controversy sometimes arises when everyday methods are touted and used for prevention or cures.

Studies regarding supplements are usually smaller in size, performed in other countries, or in private doctor's offices. When larger human studies are undertaken, patients are often receiving multiple modalities of treatment, such as drugs in tandem with supplements. This prevents the effects of the supplement alone, from being realized.

One example occurred with turkey tail mushrooms. In June 2012, *Natural Health* magazine posted an article explaining that Turkey tail mushrooms stimulate anti-tumor messengers with few side effects, unless you are allergic to mushrooms. The study was done on patients also receiving chemo and it was in Asia. I wondered if there had been any studies on women that did not have a diagnosis of cancer, for control purposes, or if there had been a study with just turkey tail mushroom treatment alone, so I looked it up.

I was surprised to find that to fill the gap between natural and science, NIH established the National Center for Complementary and Alternative Medicine (www.nccam.nih.gov) in 1991 (originally named the Office of Alternative Medicine). This branch of NIH conducted a three-year trial from 2004 to 2007 which concluded that turkey tail mushrooms are an effective adjunct to conventional chemotherapeutic medicines and radiation therapy.

Natural sources, including turkey tail mushrooms, are unlikely to be patentable, which deters big pharmaceutical companies from conducting costly clinical studies. But NIH can still do these studies. My research left me wondering why NIH did not isolate turkey tail mushrooms without chemotherapy drugs. That just doesn't seem very scientific. I am pretty sure they could find some women with breast cancer and I am pretty sure they could find some women willing to undergo treatment with turkey tail, instead of chemo.

FDA and Protecting Supplement Use

The only reason why I bring up the FDA is because preventative methods used by many people across the US may be threatened. The FDA is the organization that regulates pharmaceuticals and some food. It appears, according to recent news articles, that there may be an upcoming change in access to natural supplements. The FDA has proposed regulation on supplements to make them against the law completely.

It would be a shame if we didn't have the freedom to have supplements available as a choice. There is research available for us to find out if supplements are safe or effective. The problem comes when supplement companies don't actually use the ingredients labeled on their product or when people do not do their research or take supplements according to the label. It would be better if there were some quality control measures for supplements.

Even if supplements were approved through the FDA, there are many concerns about the current FDA approval rules and processes. One concern is when there is no cure for a disease, it takes too long for the approval process. For patients waiting for an option, this can mean pain and suffering and even death. The other concern is that states are not allowed to approve drugs independent of the FDA i.e. medical marijuana. Although at the time of this writing 20 states have legalized it for medical use and two for recreational use, so this might be changing. The third, and most relevant to supplements, is cost. Most small businesses cannot afford to put a drug or supplement through the FDA process. It costs millions of dollars.

Because of the cost involved in making and then passing drugs through the FDA, drug companies have been found to falsify data in seeking approval. The FDA has actually found fourteen cases with falsified data. Dozens of drugs were recalled or suspended due to this. There's a lesson learned here. You can't always trust a drug just because it is FDA approved.

In 1994, the Dietary Supplement Health and Education Act (DSHEA) mandated that the FDA regulate dietary supplements as foods, rather than as drugs. Since this act was established, supplements are not subject to safety and efficacy testing and there are no approval requirements.

The FDA can only take action against a dietary supplement only after they are proven to be unsafe. Manufacturers are permitted to make specific claims of health benefits, referred to as *structure or function claims* on their labels. They may not claim to treat, diagnose, cure or prevent disease and must include a disclaimer on the label.

What if there was a supplement that could cure or prevent disease? There is no place for approval of supplements for cures even if they are scientifically proven, unless the supplement company is well-funded. This seems a sad shame. As you have seen, some supplements have gotten FDA approval, which at least means they will not be taken off the market.

There are websites that help close this gap between policy and safety. At www.naturalstandard.com, www.naturaldatabase.com or www.consumerlab.com supplements are given a rating based on the scientific research and case histories available. This provides a way for people to more easily assess their scientific risk/benefit for taking a supplement. However, some of these types of sites require membership and payment. It would be great if we could have a non-profit organization evaluate supplements and have this information available to the public for free. If only the FDA would charge less for the approval process, then it might make sense for supplements to be processed through the FDA.

Dr. Joseph Mercola and Dr. Jonathan Wright point out some verbiage in the 1994 act that the FDA is now interpreting differently. The FDA believes that "new dietary supplements" must be regulated similarly to synthetic food preservatives. This is in direct violation of DSHEA which classifies supplements as food additives. If this new interpretation becomes the new norm, 80% of supplements will be taken off the market and the cost of supplements will go sky high due to the new process.

We already have an example with vitamin B6. Since 2006, there has been a controversy about the FDA (in coordination with a patent medicine company) wanting to ban the supplement form of B6 (Pyridoxal-5-Phosphate) and give the rights to this big pharmaceutical company. That new B6 approved drug will be renamed "Pyridorin", except it is the same exact molecule that is in B6.

According to the Alliance for Natural Health (ANH), the FDA has removed Pyridoxamine, which is a natural form of B6 supplements, from the market. This company would like to use Pyridoxamine in a prescription drug and has petitioned the FDA to protect its interests. Has there been a problem with B6? Has the FDA proven fraudulence? The answer is no.

I recently found out about a local attorney by the name of Jonathan W. Emord, Esq. He has fought the FDA eight times regarding supplements and won. The gist of what he does is, when the FDA requires a supplement company prove efficacy, he will argue against it in court. According to the Dietary Supplement Health and Education Act or DSHEA, supplement companies do not have to prove anything. It is the FDA that must prove fraudulence first.

It is with this existing regulatory controversy, that we can gain the understanding that pharmaceutical companies cannot ever make 100% natural products, and 100% natural products cannot always follow the same rules as pharmaceuticals. It isn't a matter of choosing sides between pharmaceutical science and natural. Doing so is limiting. There is a place for both pharmaceutical and natural methodologies in our society and that *is* okay.

As a free society, we should have the choice to utilize any methods we desire. At the same time, it is good to have systems in place to evaluate these choices for safety. Achieving balance between protection and choice is a difficult task, but the responsibility lies with the people to keep it in check. If we, as a people, do not keep a close watch over our governing bodies, these freedoms could be taken away, as has been done so many times throughout history.

We Can!

It is my hope that as we are armed with this information about proestros and breast cancer, we will pass it through each other's hands, so that we all may have a chance to help people prevent breast cancer. After we have completed the S.L.E.E.P. Method and have our hormones in balance, we can make a difference in many other areas.

The future can look better if we can slowly turn our focus about breast cancer to prevention. There are many non-profit organizations that focus on breast cancer cures and breast cancer aid for survivors. These are indeed necessary, but there are not as many groups that focus on prevention. I identified one organization (www.breastcancerfund.org) with a focus on reducing environmental contributors to breast cancer. Still, there are others that focus on single aspects such as Vitamin D, exercise or healthy eating. It would be great if there were one organization that incorporates all breast cancer prevention methods. Utilizing organizations like these to convey the truth about scientifically-backed methods, could drastically change the course of breast cancer.

Another thing we can do is we can start a documentary. We can contribute to a database of individuals who have healed or prevented breast cancer using these methods and publicize it for people to read. I hope my website, www.proestrofree.com, will be one to offer this documentary.

We can start trends. We can review this book on Amazon, Kobo or B&N so others can benefit from your opinions. We can sign our names to this book and pass it on for another reader to sign. We can start Facebook pages and share the book or foundation on our favorite social media outlet. We can do YouTube videos telling our stories of prevention.

Most importantly we can get our young women and daughters doing these steps early. If they knew the L.E.E. steps, they may never have to take supplements or creams.

We can push for more products without proestros. We can use our purchasing power to keep skin care products and cooking and food containers proestro free. We can also use our purchasing power to keep organic prices low and increase demand for pesticide free food.

Here are some other things we can do:

1. Push to get insurance companies to provide coverage for thermography and hormone testing.
2. Keep track of FDA over-reach in regards to supplements.
3. Start a non-profit that monitors and reviews supplements for the public.
4. Push to reduce pesticide use and/or to test for and add filters to our water.
5. Call local water authority and ask to eliminate fluoride and reduce chlorine in the water.
6. Get iodine back in bread and salt.
7. Become active in the GMO food fight.
8. Push pharmaceutical companies to make natural hormone patches for birth control.
9. Purchase proestro free products. Make sure companies who utilize the pink ribbon are using proestro free products.

Some way, somehow we must spread the news that most of breast cancer is caused or affected by proestros. You can do your friend or neighbor a favor by telling them about this information. It is our greatest purpose in life to help others and here is our opportunity to make a difference.

APPENDIX A: OTHER STATEGIES

Breast cancer can be prevented by addressing it from many different angles. For those trying to prevent recurrence and not diagnosed with estrogen receptor-positive breast cancer, there is still hope. A few supplements in the S.L.E.E.P. method can help due to their ability to wake up genes that are used to fight against cancer, notably curcumin and TMG. Other supplements such as olive leaf, coriolus mushroom, garlic and/or Vitamin C can help with immunity. Still others can help reduce inflammation. I have included some information here about supplements and other strategies that are known to help with breast cancer prevention. I have also included those that are known to *not* help.

Alpha-lipoic acid is a naturally occurring molecule in animal and plant cells and is a potent antioxidant. Many studies have been performed relating to diabetes. There is strong evidence it helps with type 2 diabetes by lowering blood sugar. It can also help with nerve damage caused by chemotherapy or type 2 diabetes.

There is no recommended dose. However, studies recommend 600 to 1200mg for diabetics as a supplement. If you have diabetes, have other issues, or are on chemotherapy, you should talk to your doctor before supplementing with alpha-lipoic acid. There may be interactions with the drugs you are taking or side effects. Side effects are uncommon, but there is a possibility of nausea, dizziness or rash. A good side effect is that alpha-lipoic acid regenerates glutathione.

Studies on breast cancer and alpha-lipoic acid have occurred between 2010 through 2013 ending with human trials. They all prove that alpha-lipoic acid arrests tumor cell growth, among other good things.

There were at least six studies on alpha-lipoic acid and the treatment of breast cancer listed on pubmed.org. The studies were performed at the cellular level, on mice and humans and all showed favorable results. It certainly would not hurt to take this supplement in small amounts. This supplement could help prevent breast cancer regardless of whether a person has estrogen dominance or not.

Astragalus is a genus of over 3000 species of herbs and shrubs. It has been used in ancient Chinese medicine to stimulate the immune system. It is also used in combination with chemotherapy to reduce adverse effects. It has been tested on animals and humans for treatment for allergies, ADHD, chronic fatigue syndrome and common cold to name a few.

Astragalus contains estrogen-like chemicals. A study in 2005 showed that astragalus can lower cortisol in pigs. Recent cellular studies in 2011 and 2015 demonstrated that astragalus can inhibit breast cancer cell growth. [390] [391] [392] [393]

Doctors are starting to recommend astragalus for breast cancer patients. Astragalus has been shown to be safe, if taken at recommended doses.

Vitamin B12
Dr. Jonathan Wright's book, *Stay Young & Sexy,* says vitamin B12 helps stimulate methylation and the anti-carcinogenic estrogen, 2-methoxyestradiol. He also indicates that 2-methoxyestradiol research shows it helps prostate, breast and ovarian cancers.

---

[390] Mao XF et al. Dec 2005 *J Anim Sci* "Effects of beta-glucan obtained from the Chinese herb Astragalus membranaceus and lipopolysaccharide challenge on performance, immunological, adrenal, and somatotopic responses of weaning pigs".
[391] Zhu J et al Apr 2015 *Naunyn Schmiedebergs Arch Pharmacol* "Effects and mechanism of flavonoids from Astragalus complanatus on breast cancer growth".
[392] Ye MN et al Dec 2011 *Zhong Xi Yi Jie He Xue Bao* "Effects of Astragalus polysaccharide on proliferation and Akt phosphorylation of the basal-like breast cancer cell line".
[393] Choi YK et al. 2014 *Mediators Inflamm* "Herbal extract SH003 suppresses tumor growth and metastasis of MD-MD-231 breast cancer cells by inhibiting STAT3-IL-6 signaling".

BreastDefend® by ecoNugenics
This supplement is an all-in-one for immune support and estrogen release. It combines eight researched ingredients into a single supplement. Based on the listed ingredients, BreastDefend should help fight infections, including bacteria and viruses, increase your white blood cell count and help rid your body of excess estrogen. The recommended dose is 4 capsules. This supplement has coriolus mushroom in it, though it is not hot water extracted, and is recommended by my doctor.

On April 22, 2015 News Medical published an article on this supplement titled "Botanical formula improves effect of tamoxifen drug in ER+ human breast cancer". Researchers at the Cancer Research Laboratory in Indiana found that this formula inhibited the growth of ER+ human breast cancer cells just as well as tamoxifen, the drug used in today's estrogen therapy. They also found that it enhanced the benefits of the drug tamoxifen when treating breast cancer. This is the latest study of four that shows positive results for fighting breast cancer. It is available without a prescription and there are no known side effects. I have included the label here:

BreastDefend® 120 capsules		
Supplement Facts		
Serving Size: 4 capsules		
Servings per Container: 30		
Amount Per Serving		% DV**
Cellular & Immune Proprietary Blend - [Quercetin, *(98% bioflavonoids), Scutellaria Barbata Leaf* Extract, Turmeric Rhizome Extract (*Curcuma longa*, BCM-95®), *Astragalus membranaceus* Root Extract]	950 mg	†
BreastDefend® Proprietary Herbally Enhanced Mushroom Blend - [Coriolus *(Trametes versicolor)*, Reishi *(Ganoderma lucidum), Phellinus linteus*]	500 mg	†
Diindolylmethane (DIM)	200 mg	†
**Percent Daily Values (%DV) are based on a 2,000 calorie diet		
† Daily Value not established		
Other Ingredients: Microcrystalline cellulose, vegetable capsule (natural vegetable cellulose, water), magnesium stearate, silicon dioxide.		
BCM-95® is a registered trademark of Dolca Biotech, LLC		

Crucera-SGS

Crucera SGS is another broccoli extract. It was recommended to me by my doctor, which is why I have listed it here. There is not much information available in regards to this supplement. The claim by one manufacturer is that it helps with detoxification of hormones. Again, I think we get the idea that broccoli is good!

Information taken from Thorne Research Products label:

CRUCERA-SGS is an advanced antioxidant formula that harnesses the chemoprotective properties of sulforaphane glucosinolate (SGS) – a natural substance from the seeds and sprouts of select broccoli varietals – for effective up-regulation of the body's natural phase II detoxification enzymes. SGS is an indirect antioxidant that provides long-lasting cell protection from free radical damage for days after being consumed.

When CRUCERA-SGS is ingested and begins breaking down in the gut, it releases sulforaphane, thereby activating the body's natural detoxification and antioxidant enzymes and protecting cells from free radical damage. Sulforaphane was identified in 1992 by researchers at Johns Hopkins University School of Medicine and is thought to be the key factor behind the many health benefits attributed to cruciferous vegetables.

Typical antioxidants, such as vitamin C, vitamin E, or beta carotene, work "directly" to neutralize free radicals and are usually only effective for approximately three hours after ingestion. As an "indirect" antioxidant, CRUCERA-SGS induces the activity of phase II detoxification enzymes, which then triggers broad-spectrum antioxidant activity that can last for several days – long after CRUCERA-SGS has been consumed.

Each capsule of CRUCERA-SGS contains 50 mg of sulforaphane glucosinolate – equivalent to eating 2 lbs. of cooked broccoli.

- *targeted chemoprotection*

- *safe up-regulation of the Phase II detoxification enzymes*

- *support for healthy vision and eyes*

- *support for a healthy cardiovascular and gastrointestinal system*

- *support for healthy joints*

Suggested Usage

Take 1 capsule one to two times daily or as recommended by a health-care practitioner.

Ingredients

One vegetarian capsule contains: Sulforaphane Glucosinolate (from Broccoli extract (seed) (Brassica oleracea italica)) 50 mg.

Other Ingredients: Hypromellose (derived from cellulose) capsule, Microcrystalline Cellulose, Calcium Laurate, Magnesium Laurate, Silicon Dioxide

Vitamin C

Vitamin C is generally thought to enhance immunity. I would agree with this, as I have been able to combat colds more effectively with vitamin C. However, studies on www.pubmed.gov show that vitamin C can interfere with breast cancer treatment. It can actually increase the rate that the cancer cells grow.

There is nothing to indicate that vitamin C will actually cause cancer, however. As long as you have had all your thermography and mammograms up to date and no indication of cancer, you should be fine to take it.

Dr. Joseph Mercola points out that a majority of vitamin C supplements are synthetic and there may be a major difference between the synthetic ones being used in the studies versus the whole-food supplements. He recommends making sure you are taking a quality whole-food vitamin supplement.

Vitamin E

400 IU of vitamin E daily supports female hormone balance. According to the *Mayo Clinic Breast Cancer Book*, there is not enough scientific evidence to recommend this as a supplementary therapy for breast cancer and high doses can interfere with chemotherapy. Therefore, a standard vitamin E dose is recommended.

Vitamin E in food sources may provide some protection against breast cancer, according to the following study: Kline K et al. *Journal of Mammary Gland Biology and Neoplasia* 2003 "Vitamin E and breast cancer prevention: Current status and future potential".

Enzymes

A doctor who has recently passed, Dr. Nicholas Gonzalez of New York, was treating cancer patients with enzymes. A study published in February 2006 in the *International Journal of Cancer* proves that the cause of HER2 protein increase is due to a defect in the enzyme transmission pathway meant to degrade these proteins.[394] These enzyme pathways are called kinases and are the key component to cell signaling, metabolic pathways, protein regulation, cellular transport and others. More than 500 kinases have been identified in the human body to date. I did not research which enzymes Dr. Gonzalez was using, or how they can be utilized using scientific knowledge about kinases, but it is an interesting study to note none-the-less.

One kinase mutation, PI3K/Akt kinase pathway (Phosphoinositide 3-kinase and erine/threonine kinase) is well studied in regards to cancer and insulin resistance.[395] This particular pathway is a signaling and storage pathway for lipid (fat) tissues. It plays a key role in cancer development. It also plays a role in resistance to chemotherapy. The inhibition of this pathway reduces breast cancer recurrence. Drugs have been developed to target this pathway to help chemotherapy resistance and help heal cancer by its self. Unfortunately, studies have shown an increase of infections when utilizing these drugs.[396] Detection of the PI3K/Akt enzymes can also be used to determine prognosis for survival.

---

[394] Li M et al. Feb 2006 *Int J Cancer* "Inefficient proteasomal-degradation pathway stabilizes AP-2alpha and activates HER-2/neu gene in breast cancer".

[395] Falasca M 2010 *Curr Pharm Des* "PI3K/Akt signaling pathway specific inhibitors: a novel strategy to sensitize cancer cells to anti-cancer drugs".

[396] Saeed R et al. Feb 2015 *Clin Cancer Res* "Higher risk of infections with PI3K-AKT-mTOR pathway inhibitors in patients with advanced solid tumors on Phase 1 clinical Trials".

A specific enzyme, the Shp2 enzyme, has been found to be upregulated in 70% of invasive breast cancers.[397] Too much of this enzyme turns off tumor suppressor genes p27 and p53. There is an experimental drug developed to turn off this enzyme, but it has only been studied in mice at this time.

These are examples where we can see real science telling us what is causing the problems (enzyme pathway overstimulation, gene mutations) and then we can find real doctors who are treating them. In effect, increase in the wrong enzymes or depletion of good enzymes can affect gene transmissions which can cause cancer growth.

You have to wonder why enzymes are overstimulated in HER2 positive patients in the first place. Perhaps it is the lack of nutritionally and enzymatically balanced food in today's diet. Here is what a colleague of mine, Linda Dulicai has to say about enzymes in diet:

"Digestive health is crucial, and enzymes are key. If we lack enzymes in our food and do not supplement, digestion suffers and constipation can be one symptom. When we are constipated, we recycle toxins again and again through our bodies. Enzymes help us digest our food, thereby reducing or alleviating constipation and toxins.

If constipation is not dealt with, our bodies act out. Certain types of cancers have been linked to chronic constipation. For example, one study shows that while having other women in the family with breast cancer increased a family member's risk by 25%, that risk could be reduced by 46% by avoiding or alleviating constipation.

If we lack enzymes in our food, we are also hindered in producing the enzymes required for basic functions. For instance, if we do not digest

---

[397] Max Delbrueck Center for Molecular Medicine (MDC) Berlin-Buch Mar 25 2015 *News Medical* "Shp2 enzyme blocks protection program, boosts tumor growth".

the fat and protein we eat, we cannot properly produce hormones. Many cancers have hormonal imbalance components.

Break the cycle of nutrition, digestion and utilization, and our bodies will then find unending ways to act out."

A practitioner for more than 38 years, Linda Dulicai is a Certified Natural Health Professional and an Advanced Loomis Digestive Health Specialist educated in more than 25 modalities of wellness. She is CEO of The Healthy Zone.

Here, we can understand how the food you eat and its nutritional components are directly related to a lack of enzymes. This lack of enzymes in turn, can affect the functionality of cells, hormones and genes.

Eradicating Chemicals and Metals
Eradicating proestros out of your life may not be easy, but it is possible and may be necessary for healing. The first thing we need to do is eradicate chemicals out of our environment. In addition to the actions in the *Eliminate* section, there may be a few other things we can do.

I recently found out that some plants may actually absorb formaldehyde and chemicals right out of the air. A few of the plants that can do this are aloe, fichus, and spider plants. It is especially helpful when the house is closed up for the winter because most plants absorb carbon dioxide and excrete oxygen. Adding a plant or two helps the air you breathe. Just keep in mind that mold can grow in the soil if you overwater or if new soil is never added or leaves collect. After you have effectively eliminated known environmental sources, you might consider utilizing your natural process to eliminate additional chemicals out of your body.

Our body has natural processes in place to guide these chemicals out. However, if your body is over-burdened with chemicals, it can halt these natural processes. There are only a few ways to know if your body is over-burdened by chemicals. Sometimes, you don't know until you are actually getting them out. You may notice differences in your stool or may have small reactions to the process such as being tired or shaky. Regardless, most people have had over accumulation of chemicals and there is no reason not to attempt to eliminate build-up of these proestros from the body. Some people have made claims that eliminating chemicals from the body by using glutathione, reduced breast cancer lumps.

Infrared Sauna

If you prefer not to use pills, patches or suppositories, you can do a physical detox using an infrared sauna. Infrared is a band of energy in the electromagnetic spectrum that has been used effectively for millennia to treat and ease certain maladies and discomforts. According to NIH, heating of the skin with FIR (Far Infrared Radiation) has been shown to help with cardiovascular conditions and diseases, lower stress and fatigue, help with cell repair and reduce pain and stiffness associated with rheumatoid arthritis and spondylitis. A 2008 study showed that FIR is effective at inhibiting cancer on five types of human cancer cells, including breast cancer.[398]

I started using an infrared sauna once per week at my doctor's office. The cost to pay per visit was about $50 per session. After a while, I decided to buy a sauna from Craig's List. It paid for itself in two months. It helps detox estrogens, heavy metals and many other chemicals. It also helps alleviate sore muscles and heal colds. I still use the sauna a few times per month during winter months.

Folate is the natural compound found in food such as green leafy vegetables. It is one of the B complex vitamins. It is important to point out that folic acid is a synthetic form of the vitamin found in supplements and is not the same as folate. Studies have been performed on both folate and folic acid and sometimes the terms are used interchangeably, but they do not have the same effects.

---

[398] Ishibashi J et al. 2008 *Med Oncol* "The effects inhibiting the proliferation of cancer cells by far-infrared radiation (FIR) are controlled by the basal expression level of heat shock protein (HSP) 70A".

It is folate's deficiency in humans that is associated with breast cancer and other cancers. Studies in 2007 in Sweden and 2011 in China showed a link between reduced risk of breast cancer and folate intake. [399] [400] The 2011 study showed a 42% reduction of hormone negative breast cancer for pre-menopausal women with average intakes of 404 micrograms per day. [401] A 2009 study at Free Hutchison Cancer Research Center showed that folate was 22% protective against estrogen receptor breast cancers in post-menopausal women and even more for estrogen receptor-negative breast cancers. [402]

In his book, Dr. Jonathan Wright mentions that folate helps with methylation and increase of 2-methoxyestradiol (2ME2), which is perhaps why it is linked with a lower breast cancer risk. A urine test will show if you are low in 2ME2 and you can decide then if you need folate. My urine test from US Biotek Labs did not test the 2ME2 hormone. However, urine hormone tests through Meridian Valley Laboratory routinely do include it. A natural metabolite form of folate, 5–methyl tetrahydrofolate (THF), has shown to increase 2ME2 even more than folate itself.

In conclusion, it may be beneficial, and definitely not harmful, to take folate. The recommended daily allowance for folate is 400mcg. Just make certain that you are using folate and not folic acid which has been linked to marginally higher levels of cancer.

Garlic can boost the immune system but it can also affect chemotherapy, so you wouldn't want to eat or utilize it during chemotherapy.

[399] Ericson U et al. Aug 2007 *Am J Clin Nutr* "High folate intake is associated with lower breast cancer incidence in postmenopausal women in the Malmo Diet and Cancer cohort".

[400] Wien TN et al. 2012 *BMJ Open* "Cancer risk with folic acid supplements: a systematic review and meta-analysis".

[401] Stuart, Dagny Sep 2011 *Research News at Vanderbilt University* "Folate may lower breast cancer risk for some".

[402] Maruti SS et al. Feb 2009 *Am J Clin Nutr* "Folate and one-carbon metabolism nutrients from supplements and diet in relation to breast cancer risk".

Green Tea Extract

The active components of green tea are the catechins which are flavan-3 oils. One of these oils, Epigallocatechin-3-gallate (EGCG), was shown to inhibit a number of tumor cell proliferation and survival pathways.[403] Green tea contains a small amount of quercetin which has been shown to have anti-cancer effects. A study of Chinese women found that daily intake of green tea had a strong effect on decreasing mammographic density.[404]

Glucoraphanin is an active component in broccoli and a precursor to sulforaphane. Sulforaphane is found in broccoli, Brussels sprouts and cabbage. It is proven in at least three animal studies on pubmed.gov to boost cell enzymes that protect against cancer causing chemicals.

Eating the vegetables themselves wouldn't give the same quantity as was done in these trials. The compound is in much higher quantities and is taken from the sprouts, not the mature broccoli plant. Here again, we see that broccoli extracts are good!

Glutathione is what your body normally uses to eliminate proestros from the body. Typically, ingesting glutathione does not give the body enough to do effective cleansing, quickly. It is broken down in the stomach before it gets anywhere in the body. Glutathione patches or suppositories are the best methods to increase glutathione levels. According to her books, Suzanne Somers uses glutathione patches regularly.

An online blogger by the name of Shirley was able to shrink her breast lumps completely by using glutathione supplementation. She used *Immunocal*, which is a dietary glutathione. You can read more about

---

[403] Thangapazham RL et al. Dec 2007 *Cancer Biol Ther* "Green tea polyphenol and epigallocatechin gallate induce apoptosis and inhibit invasion in human breast cancer cells">

[404] Wu AH et al. 2008 *Cancer Epidemiolo Biomarkers Prev* "Green tea, soy and mammographic density in Singapore Chinese women".

her testimony at www.shirleys-wellness-cafe.com/women/breastcancer.aspx.

I3C is the pre-cursor to DIM. Although there have been many studies indicating its success to treat breast cancer, it has actually promoted breast cancer growth in some studies. In 1995, a study was published that showed that I3C increased 2-OHE1 formation, which is known as a protective marker in breast cancer. [405]

In 2000 Dr. MC Bell and team performed cervical biopsies after 12 weeks on participants with cervical intraepithelial neoplasia. They found 47% (8/17) who took I3C had a complete regression. The precancerous growths disappeared! This was a "gold standard" trial which was double blind and placebo controlled. Doses up to 300 and 400 mg were used with no side effects.[406]

There are issues related to absorption of I3C, so typically, high doses are given. High doses are associated with side effects and toxicity. [407] You are better off taking DIM directly.

Inflammation Reduction
There are several reasons why the body may cause an inflammatory reaction using inflammation. If you have food allergies or food sensitivities, this can be a trigger. Lack of vitamin D can be another. Certain bacteria, allergies or viruses can also cause inflammation.

Because we know inflammation can be a contributor to breast cancer growth, it would be a good idea to do food allergy testing to rule out food sensitivities. Some metals are known to cause inflammation, so having a metals test is another good idea. Lastly, some bacteria such as

---

[405] Bradlow HL et al. Oct 1995 *Environ Health Prospect* "Effects of pesticides on the ratio of 16 alpha/2-hydroxyestrone: a biologic marker of breast cancer risk".
[406] Bell MC et al. Aug 2000 *Gynecol Oncol* "Placebo-controlled trial of indole-3-carbinol in the treatment of CIN".
[407] Arneson DW et al. 2001 Am Assoc Cancer Res "Pharmacokinetics of 3-3 – Diindolylmethane following oral administration of Indole-3-carbinol to human subjects".

Lyme disease can cause significant inflammation. If you think there is a possibility you could have contracted Lyme through a tick or other parasite, it would be good to confirm and address it. Reducing inflammation after finding out you have food allergies, Lyme disease or high metals may take a long time, but there are other things you can do to reduce inflammation overall.

Vitamin D reduces inflammation significantly and there are even drugs and other supplements such as boswellia and *Flexacill* that help reduce inflammation.

Vitamin K2, K3 There are not that many studies on vitamin K and breast cancer. Approximately 19 studies are on Vitamin K3 and its effect on breast cancer which are showing promising results for fighting cancer. Vitamin K3 derivatives (specifically CR108) have been shown to inhibit cancer growth on both HER-2 and non-HER-2 expressed cancer cells. There are no clinical trials on this as of yet. Scientists say there may be hope to use this in conjunction with chemotherapy in the future. Nothing was studied on the use of K3 as a preventative except for prevention of bone loss due to cancer. Plumbagin, a vitamin K2 analogue, is known as a toxin. K2 doses of up to 45mg/day appeared safe in one study.

Liver Detox
Many people I know, including myself, have also tried liver detox. I found it to be fairly aggressive because it involves fasting for a whole day and drinking lots of olive oil and lemon juice. It is difficult to get all these liquids down and it made my stomach queasy. I was unable to find the science to back this method, but there were definite visible results in the stool that are comparable to pictures of gall bladder contents after removal.

Methylsulfonylmethane (MSM) increases your supply of this methyl group, which may contribute to raising your 2ME2. Stress uses up the methyl groups in order to make adrenaline. If you don't feel like taking another supplement, reducing stress can make more methyl groups available.

MSM has been shown to substantially decrease the viability of breast cancer cells in cellular and mouse studies. It effectively targets the major molecules involved in tumor development, progression and metastasis. This was also true for triple-negative receptors, which is great news for ladies who do not test estrogen positive.[408]

Although the toxicity of this methyl group is reported as low, more testing will need to be done in humans to find the right dose and possible side effects.[409]

Magnesium Sulfate improves efficiency of iodine treatment. It is not known why.

Mushrooms are being used more and more for breast cancer prevention. Turkey Tail mushroom has shown good potential with testing at NIH. If NIH would test it without chemo, then we would have the science to back it up.

Another mushroom is getting high marks for breast cancer prevention by increasing white blood cell count. This mushroom has been in use as folk medicine for a long time. Today, Japan is using this mushroom in IV bags for women undergoing chemotherapy. This mushroom is called the coriolus mushroom. It is also called *PSK* and that term has been copyrighted.

The key to coriolus is that it must be hot water extracted so that the polysaccharides are present. This mushroom has been studied and peer reviewed. The only company using hot water extraction in the US is *Mushroom Science* (www.mushroomscience.com). Katherine Albrecht

---

[408] Lim EJ et al. 2012 *PLoS One* "Methylsulfonylmethane suppresses breast cancer growth by down-regulating STAT3 and STAT5b pathways".
[409] Parcell S. Feb 2002 *Altern Med Rev* "Sulfur in human nutrition and applications in medicine".

is a nationally syndicated radio host, author and breast cancer survivor who is using this coriolus mushroom to prevent future breast cancer. She details information about this mushroom in a blog. Here is her testimonial:

How I survived my cancer treatments with coriolus mushroom (Katherine's true story).

After my intense two-year battle with Stage IIIC breast cancer, I'm a big believer in chemotherapy, radiation, and other "conventional" treatments. They have improved my odds of living out my natural lifespan from 1%-2% to still living and breathing today, which you'll have to admit is a big improvement. But as you know, conventional therapy can be very hard on the body. One solution is to find natural, food-based solutions that have been scientifically shown to help mitigate the side effects of cancer treatment. One of the lifesaver supplements I took during my cancer treatment—and will take daily for the rest of my life—is coriolus mushroom.

Coriolus helps the body deal naturally with a major treatment side effect of chemotherapy called neutropenia — a drop in white blood cell count that occurs a few days after a chemotherapy infusion. Chemo works by destroying fast-dividing cells, and because that impacts white blood cells (the body's immune cells) that leaves you vulnerable to infection and illness.

Before each chemo treatment, my oncologist would check my white blood cell count. If it was too low, they would delay or even discontinue chemotherapy. So by keeping my white blood cell count up, I could increase the chances of completing my chemotherapy regimen, which increased my odds of killing the cancer — and surviving. Initially, I experienced this awful cycle. After each infusion of chemo, my white blood cell count would drop way low, and I would become a magnet for infection. I once got so sick from a bronchial infection that I couldn't breathe and one night almost checked myself into the emergency room at 2:00 AM.

"Conventional medicine" deals with this drop in white blood cells by administering a $3000 drug called Neulasta (or Neupogen), which forces your bone marrow to produce white blood cells. Shortly after each chemo, I had to go back to the hospital to get this hugely expensive — and painful — shot. Because Neulasta works by forcing the bone marrow to produce white blood cells, it hurts deep in your bones, so you may need additional pain medication. This cycle of needing drugs (pain meds) to handle the drugs (Neulasta) to handle the drugs (chemo) that you need to handle the cancer is a bit crazy.

Then my wonderful husband did some research and discovered that coriolus mushroom could help me escape that vicious cycle. In Japan, they've found that an inexpensive, natural coriolus extract boosts the white blood cell count tremendously, so over there they skip the $3,000 Neulasta shot and all the side effects. They've purified it into a drug called PSK which they deliver in IV bags right at the chemo center.

Cancer centers here in America won't give you an IV infusion of PSK, but you can take the mushroom in pills yourself. If my own experience is any indication, it works like a charm. My husband tracked down the only US seller of properly extracted, PSK-grade coriolus: Mushroom Science's Coriolus Super Strength PSK Formula.

We ordered six bottles (and got one free), and I took four capsules daily throughout my cancer treatment. My oncologist was fine with my taking it, since it's essentially just food.

The amazing part is that these simple mushroom pills quickly boosted my white blood cell count back to the normal range to where I no longer needed Neulasta. My white counts were so normal that my oncologist was quite surprised. More importantly, I stopped catching every infection under the sun after every chemo treatment, and that meant I could continue letting the chemo do its life-saving work.

But it gets even better. It turns out that coriolus not only protects your immune system through chemo, but researchers have been testing whether it might fight cancer in its own right. There's at least one FDA-approved trial going on right now in the USA for breast cancer. The

results are pretty compelling. Check out the peer-reviewed medical studies at PubMed:
http://www.ncbi.nlm.nih.gov/pubmed?term=coreolus%20psk%20chemotherapy

It's been almost a year since my last chemo treatment, and I continue to take coriolus daily. (We buy it by the case.) As long as I can continue to afford it, and Mushroom Science keeps selling it, I will take it daily for the rest of my life.

One more thing – we did a lot of research before selecting Mushroom Science as our supplier. They are the only producer of coriolus that uses the HOT WATER EXTRACT method, which is the only preparation method for coriolus clinically tested and shown to work. The cheap coriolus sold by other suppliers is a ground up powder of the mushroom mycelium (the stringy fibers underneath the mushroom), which is super cheap, but does not have the same polysaccharide composition. Since the polysaccharides in the coriolus are what make it work, I'm sticking to the hot water version.

I reached out to the Mushroom Science guys for a discount, since I buy so much from them and I am such a believer in what they do. They offered me a coupon code I can pass on. It's the word "Katherine". If you use it, they will send you a free book on the medicinal benefits of mushrooms.

N-Acetyl-L Cysteine
Acetylcystein (also known as N-acetylcysteine or N-Acetyl-L Cystein or NAC) is a supplement primarily used when treating overdose of acetaminophen. The primary claim of this compound is that it protects the liver and serves as an antioxidant. Since we are already protecting the liver with milk thistle, NAC may not be necessary.

However, after age 35 we stop producing glutathione so it would be a good protective supplement. NAC is a precursor to glutathione. Glutathione prevents free radical damage from toxic exposures. It is excellent for detoxifying the intestines. According to Dr. William LaValley from Austin, TX, low doses of this supplement should be fine to ingest.[410] A mouse study in 2007 at the University of VA showed that large doses of NAC can cause damage to heart and lungs.[411]

200 to 500mg once per day is probably okay in most non-cancer cases.

It can be also used as a cough medicine because it breaks the bonds in mucus, making it easier to cough up.

There have not been many studies of NAC and breast cancer. One Russian study in 2012 performed using metformin and NAC, showed that NAC can reduce breast density.[412] Since lowering breast density can perhaps lower breast cancer risk, this is a possible association and helpful supplement.

Using NAC while detoxifying from mercury is not a good idea because it could interfere with the detoxification process. NAC is available in foods like spinach and Brussels sprouts. If you eat these often, you should not need to take this supplement.

Poly-MVA is an alpha-lipoic acid with palladium. It is a natural chemotherapeutic agent. Its effectiveness depends on the stage of cancer. If treating cancer, it should be administered by a doctor for proper use.

Probiotics help maintain a healthy digestive system. They help eliminate proestros and excess estrogens in the intestines and help immunity as well. What good is it if we are constipated and can't get

---

[410] www.mercola.com Sept 2007 "This Common Antioxidant Supplement Could Cause You Loads of Trouble".

[411] Palmer LA et al. 2007 *J Clin Invest* "S-Nitrosothiols signal hypoxia-mimetic vascular pathology".

[412] Bershtein DA et al. 2012 *Vopr Onkol* "N-acetylcysteine compares favorably to metformin on mammographic density in postmenopausal women".

these proestros out? If you eat a healthy diet, rich in vegetables and fermented foods such as yogurt, you may not need to take a probiotic.

If you do choose to use a probiotic, the quality is of utmost importance. Many probiotics once swallowed, never make it to the intestines. There are a few name brands that I have used that appear to work for me. They are *Integrative Therapeutics, Pearls", Bio-Kult, Axe Naturals LIVE Probiotics, Garden of Life Primal Defense* and Dr. Joseph Mercola's *Complete Probiotics*.

Quercetin is a plant pigment found in fruits, vegetables, leaves and grains. The most common foods it is found in are dill, red onion, buckwheat, sweet potato, red delicious apples, organic tomatoes and broccoli.

There have been many studies on quercetin at the cellular level and a few on mice. In these studies, it has shown to help with asthma, cancer, eczema, fibromyalgia, hypertension, inflammation and as a potential antiviral. It has not been approved for any health claims yet by the FDA since there are no tests or case studies on humans.

One problem associated with quercetin seems to be its bioavailability (absorbability) to the body. One study with rats in 2008 demonstrated 69% of it was excreted through the urine.[413] This indicates a low retention and high excretion rate.

I found two 2013 studies showing quercetin's anti-growth effect on breast cancer cells. Both studies demonstrate that quercetin inhibits growth in breast cancer cells in multiple ways.[414] [415] A third study in 2014 has found a way to make quercetin more bioavailable using it as

---

[413] Mullen W et al. Dec 2008 *J Agric Food Chem* "Bioavailability of [2-(14) C] quercetin-4'-glucoside in rats".

[414] Deng XH et al. Nov 2013 *Exp Ther Med* "Effects of quercetin o the proliferation of breast cancer cells and expression of surviving in vitro".

[415] Chen FP et al. Dec 2013 *Climacteric* "Phytoestrogens induce apoptosis through a mitochondria/caspase pathway in human breast cancer cells".

Q-NLC.[416] Using it in this altered state dramatically enhanced the anti-cancer activities and availability to cancer cells. I have a feeling we will be seeing more of this Q-NLC!

Since these studies have been at the cellular level, there is no recommended dosage. However, low levels have shown to not have any side effects in mice. There may be interactions with some antibiotics such as fluoroquinolones, so make sure you check with your doctor before taking this.

S-Adenosylmethionine (SAM-e) is a methyl donor that naturally raises your 2ME2 levels. Since TMG increases SAM-e, you would not need to take this in addition to TMG.

Selenium is a naturally occurring substance in our body but is only found in trace amounts in food and soil. There are over 300 published studies on Selenium. 200 to 400 mcg per day is the recommended dose. If you are taking an ingested iodine supplement, you may want to take the higher dose of selenium. Selenium helps absorption of iodine into your body's cells.

Studies and case reports show selenium inhibits premalignant breast cell growth and tumor incidence after exposure to carcinogens. G. Rowan, Ph.D., an associate professor at Tulane University, found that selenium "inhibits receptor function in breast cancer cells".

Trans-pterostilbebe is an anti-oxidant found primarily in blueberries. A study in 2014, showed that pterostilbebe was able to induce apoptosis in both, estrogen negative and estrogen positive breast cancer cells, however the apoptosis was much higher in the estrogen negative cells. [417]

---

[416] Sun M et al. Jan 2014 *Colloids Surf B Biointerfaces* "Quercetin-nanostructured lipid carriers: Characteristics and anti-breast cancer activities in vitro".
[417] Pan C et al. Aug 2014 *PLoS One* "Estrogen Receptor-α36 Is Involved in Pterostilbene-Induced Apoptosis and Anti-Proliferation in In Vitro and In Vivo Breast Cancer".

This is great news for those with estrogen negative breast cancer. There are approximately 22 studies on this ingredient and breast cancer, but none on humans. There are plenty of supplements available with this ingredient in it at this time, although there is not enough research on people to recommend it in high doses. Blueberries are a key food to eat to get this nutrient into the body!

Trans-Resveratrol is a grape/red wine derivative that has been the subject of numerous scientific studies and is showing promise in lowering risks from cancer to cardiovascular disease. Nutrition experts recommend a dose of between 50 to 250 mg per day. Too bad a glass of red wine only has .02 to 2.0 mg per glass. Wouldn't it be nice if all we needed to do was drink a glass of red wine every day?

The researchers from the Faculty of Pharmacy at the University of Calabria in Italy report that resveratrol blocks the effect of estrogen and can prevent malignant growth of breast cancer in women when they directly tested resveratrol on breast cancer cells.[418] Another study in 2013 in Taiwan had the same finding for genistein, resveratrol and quercetin.[415]

Vinegar foot pads or baths is another method used for detoxing. The water or foot baths turn dark grey when this method is being used which may be an indication of metals and toxins being released. This may also be beneficial, but there is not enough scientific data to show the benefit and quantity of chemicals removed doing vinegar detox.

XenoProtX by Xymogen
This product is exclusively patented and has at least 15 substances that have at least some scientific proof to aid in the elimination of estrogen or prevent breast cancer. I have listed the supplements below that are in the formula, some of which are in Step S, i.e. DIM and Calcium-D-

---

[418] Phillip J Oct 2011 www.naturalnews.com "Resveratrol lowers breast cancer risk by estrogen growth factor".

Glucarate. The problem with an all-in-one approach for detoxing is that the amount of each supplement may not be enough to adequately provide the desired effect. The other thing with this supplement is that it contains magnesium stearate, which may affect absorption of the actual ingredients.

This could be a good maintenance supplement to take after you have completed a full estrogen detoxification program. You can take two capsules of this per day and get all these great supplements.

XenoProtX™
Comprehensive Support for Detoxification*
Share
XenoProtX™ is a comprehensive formula designed to support phase I and phase II liver detoxification of environmental pollutants, endocrine disruptors, estrogen metabolites, xenoestrogens, and other toxins. XenoProtX also supports antioxidant activity throughout the detoxification process. Micronutrients, phytonutrients, and activated cofactors provide additional support for energy production, cellular protection, and liver function during crucial metabolic biotransformation processes. *

SUPPLEMENT FACTS
Serving Size: 2 Capsules

	Amount Per Serving	% Daily Value
Folate (as 6(S)-5-methyltetrahydrofolic acid, glucosamine salt†)	*200 mcg*	*50%*
Selenium (as methylselenocysteine)	*15 mcg*	*21%*
Calcium-D-Glucarate	*250 mg*	****
Green Tea Aqueous Extract (Camellia sinensis) (leaf)⬚(80% polyphenols, 60% catechins, 30% EGCG, 6% caffeine)	*250 mg*	****

Glucoraphanin (from broccoli extract) (Brassica oleracea italica) (seed)(SGS™)	15 mg	**
Alpha-Lipoic Acid	100 mg	**
N-Acetyl-L-Cysteine	100 mg	**
Milk Thistle Extract (Silybum marianum)⬚(seed) (80% silymarin)	100 mg	**
DIM (diindolylmethane)	75 mg	**
Quercetin (as quercetin dihydrate) (from Dimorphandra mollis) (bud)	50 mg	**
Turmeric Extract (Curcuma longa) (rhizome) (95% curcuminoids)	50 mg	**
trans-Resveratrol (as Polygonum cuspidatum root extract)	18.5 mg	**
trans-Pterostilbene (pTeroPure®)	15.5 mg	**
Siberian and Dahurian Larch Tree Extract (Larix dahurica)⬚(Larix sibirica) (Larix gmelinii) (sawlogs) (90% dihydroquercetin) (FlavitPURE™)	5.5 mg	**
Black Pepper Extract (Piper nigrum) (fruit)(BioPerine®)	5 mg	**

** Daily Value not established.

All XYMOGEN® Formulas Meet or Exceed cGMP Quality Standards.

RESOURCES

Books

Breast Cancer: Risks and Prevention Fourth Edition Angela Lanfranchi, M.D., F.A.C.S and Joel Brind, Ph.D. 2005, 2007

Dr. John Lee's Hormone Balance Made Simple John R. Lee, M.D. and Virginia Hopkins 2006

Dr. Mercola's Total Health Program Dr. Joseph Mercola, 2003-2005

Dr. Susan Love's Breast Book Susan M. Love, M.D. 2010

Endocrine-Disrupting Chemicals: An Endocrine Society Scientific Statement Evanthia Diamanti-Kandarakis, Jean-Pierre Bourguignon, Linda C Giudice, Russ Hauser, Gail S Prins, Ana M Soto, R Thomas Zeller and Adrea C Gore June 2009

Gut and Psychology Syndrome Dr. Natasha Campbell-McBride, M.D. 2010

I'm Too Young for This Suzanne Somers 2013

Internal Bliss Dr. Natasha Campbell McBride, 2010

Iodine Why You Need It Why You Can't Live Without It David Brownstein, M.D., 2009

Knockout Interviews with Doctors Who Are Curing cancer" Suzanne Somers 2009

Stay Young & Sexy with Bio-Identical Hormone Replacement Jonathan V. Wright, M.D., Lane Lenard, Ph.D., 2010

Surviving Triple-Negative Breast Cancer Patricia Prijatel, 2013

The Breast Cancer Prevention Diet Dr. Bob Arnot, 1998

The Breast Cancer Epidemic: 10 facts A Patrick Sneider II et al. The Linacre Quarterly 81 (3) 2014

Healing Breast Cancer Naturally Veronique Desaulniers

The Mayo Clinic Breast Cancer Book Lynn C. Hartmann, M.D., Charles L Loprinzi, M.D., 2012

The Natural Prostate Cure Roger Mason, 2000 p18

Tox-Sick Suzanne Somers, 2015

Waking the Warrior Goddess Christine Horner

The Whole-Food Guide for Breast Cancer Survivors Edward Bauman, M.D. M.ED., Ph.D., Helayne Waldman, MS EDD, 2012

What Your Doctor May Not Tell You about Breast Cancer John R. Lee, M.D., David Zava, Ph.D. and Virginia Hopkins, 2002

Websites

www.pubmed.org

www.breastcancer.org

www.breastcancerfund.org

www.mayoclinic.org

ww5.komen.org

www.tahomaclinic.com

www.mercola.com

www.wellnessmama.com

www.hakalalabs.com

www.grassrootshealth.net

www.lef.org

www.thinkbeforeyoupink.org

www.healthywomen.org

www.epa.gov

www.cancer.org

www.consumerreports.org

www.usgs.gov

www.cornandsoybeandigest.com

http://water.usgs.gov

http://pubs.usgs.gov

http://onlinelibrary.wiley.com

www.seer.com

http://www.ncbi.nlm.nih.gov

www.fda.gov

www.drwilson.com

www.drsircus.com

www.centerforsaferwireless.us

www.proestrofree.com

Organizations

Think Before You Pink (www.thinkbeforeyoupink.org) is a national breast cancer organization that does "not accept funding from entities that profit or contribute to cancer including the pharmaceutical companies". One of the great things it does is verify that companies using pink ribbons as marketing tools are not using toxic chemicals in their products that cause cancer or are developing cancer drugs themselves.

45842174R00208

Made in the USA
Middletown, DE
15 July 2017